"Relax the body, clear the mind, and act against what you foolishly fear. That's how to free yourself from anxiety. This book describes how to do it. Greiner-Ferris and Khalsa blend a pleasant yoga relaxation program with Eastern wisdom and cognitive behavioral ways of knowing and doing that interested readers can easily follow to free themselves from needless anxieties and lead an enlightened life."

—**Bill Knaus, EdD**, author of *The Cognitive Behavioral Workbook for Anxiety*

"Greiner-Ferris and Khalsa build on years of evidence to present their readers with a six-week program to reduce anxiety. *The Yoga-CBT Workbook for Anxiety* is filled with great ideas for decreasing anxiety and living a more productive life! The step-by-step yoga, meditation, and cognitive behavioral therapy (CBT) strategies are practical, straightforward, and helpful. I highly recommend this book for anyone who experiences anxiety, is a mental health provider, or is a yoga practitioner or teacher."

—**Ellen Tuchman, PhD**, associate professor and coordinator of the Evidence-Based Mental Health Project at the New York University Silver School of Social Work

"Julie Greiner-Ferris and Manjit Kaur Khalsa have created a breakthrough approach to treating anxiety with *The Yoga-CBT Workbook for Anxiety*. This workbook presents a seamless integration of researched, cutting-edge mind-body techniques and traditional therapeutic approaches. These techniques are for everyone, and illustrate that the mind-body connection is the most powerful way to address both the mental and physical aspects of anxiety."

—**Hari Kaur Khalsa**, author of *A Woman's Book of Meditation*, coauthor of *A Woman's Book of Yoga*, and Kundalini yoga teacher, trainer, and owner at Hari NYC

"Blending yoga and CBT is genius. The transformation among my clients has been significant. As a clinician who runs yoga-CBT groups, this workbook is invaluable for clients to keep their practice going. The workbook is clear, concise, and informative. It's a must-have for clients and clinicians alike."

—**Jacqueline Vorpahl, PhD**, owner and child and family psychologist at Vorpahl Psychology Associates, LLC, and creator of the Chilloutz app for kids

GW00683704

"I found the neurobiology involved in a person's anxiety, and in how to take control over that anxiety, to be described very clearly and thoroughly in *The Yoga-CBT Workbook for Anxiety*, especially for a nonscientific layperson-. Who knew that carbon dioxide plays such an important role in our thoughts, emotions, and behavior? Therapeutic principles of treating many psychiatric conditions were well incorporated into this guide. Particularly valuable is that this workbook goes beyond illustrating how to decrease symptoms; it takes the reader to the next level: how anxiety impacts a person's communication and relationships. Understanding the biochemical processes that are involved in one's feelings of self-worth and one's ability to communicate is only one part of the 'equation.' Integrating that knowledge with meditation and yoga techniques can produce changed behavior. Incorporating the guiding principles set forth in this workbook can lead to a richer, better, and calmer quality of life."

> —**Dallas R. Gulley, LICSW**, assistant vice president of Behavioral Health Services Division at Riverside Community Care

"This workbook represents an important contribution to the self-help literature on managing anxiety. The authors, both seasoned clinicians, started with a clinical intervention that they developed and utilized with many clients, then conducted research that demonstrated its effectiveness. From that foundation, they have crafted a self-guided tool and imbued it with clarity and compassion. That tool can help people manage the problematic anxiety that all too often interferes with living. Much is written about integrating mind and body; this self-help workbook succeeds. Both yoga and CBT are made accessible, and a six-week path of physical and cognitive steps is simply and effectively laid out to help. I highly recommend it!"

> —**Jon Jaffe, LICSW**, vice president of Consultation and Behavioral Health Divisions at the May Institute

The YOGA-CBT WORKBOOK for Anxiety

Total Relief for Mind & Body

JULIE GREINER-FERRIS, LICSW

MANJIT KAUR KHALSA, EdD

New Harbinger Publications, Inc.

Note to Reader

All case material and clinical examples in this book are fictionalized and are not a representation of any specific individual person.

Medical Disclaimer

While yoga practices are empowering and safe, they are not substitutes for medical care. The benefits attributed to the practice of Kundalini Yoga as taught by Yogi Bhajan® stem from centuries-old yogic tradition; results will vary with individuals. Sometimes yoga practices are most effective as supplemental self-care to counseling and medical advice.

Professional treatment, including medications, can be helpful, especially if you have a history of trauma, depression, or a diagnosed anxiety disorder. If you are receiving treatment for anxiety, please consult with your therapist or doctor before using the practices in the book. As with any physical exercise, if you have any physical health conditions, consult with your medical provider before attempting the yoga in this book.

Copyright © 2017 by Julie Greiner-Ferris and Manjit Kaur Khalsa
New Harbinger Publications, Inc.
5674 Shattuck Avenue
Oakland, CA 94609
www.newharbinger.com

Acquisitions Editors: Melissa Valentine and Elizabeth Hollis Hansen; KRI Editor: Siri Neel Kaur Khalsa; Developmental Editor: Gretel Hakanson; Line Editor: Hannah Benoit; Copy Editor: Marisa Solís; Photographer: David S. Marshall; Model: Kathryn Greiner-Ferris

---

Library of Congress CIP on file

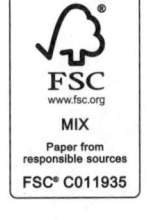
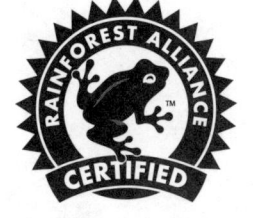

19   18   17

10   9   8   7   6   5   4   3   2   1   First Printing

Contents

INTRODUCTION

Toward a Calmer Way of Being

All of us experience some anxiety from time to time, just as we all feel joy, anger, sorrow, love, and the whole range of human emotion. It is virtually impossible to go throughout life without feeling anxious at some point—at times it can be fleeting, other times debilitating. When anxiety is overpowering, it can feel as if your life has been derailed—a variety of uncomfortable symptoms often follows in its wake, leaving you believing that anxiety is utterly unmanageable.

It's not.

This book will teach you how to effectively deal with problematic anxiety so that you can get your life back!

What is anxiety? In the simplest terms, it is your reaction to something that frightens you. Anxiety can be caused by a current experience or situation, or it can be triggered by a thought or a stimulus, such as a certain smell or sight, that reminds you of a frightening event from your past. Whatever its trigger, the fear response created by anxiety has a dramatic effect on your thoughts and your physical state.

A variety of biochemical changes in your body, fueled by your memories and imagination, combine to produce the tense and agitated sensation we call anxiety. Having this sensation can be so overwhelming that it can affect how you go about your life—how you interact with others, your avoidance of places or situations, how you treat yourself, your interpretation of future and past events, and so on.

You may have developed habits to keep your anxiety under control, but maybe they're no longer working. Or maybe they've never worked very well. Moving beyond current psychological thought, the *Yoga-CBT Workbook for Anxiety* offers a new approach to managing your symptoms of anxiety. Yoga–cognitive behavioral therapy (Y-CBT) teaches you to quiet your mind and your body simultaneously by blending the methods of cognitive behavioral therapy (CBT) with yogic philosophies and techniques (Y). The result is a comprehensive and transformational resolution of anxiety symptoms.

Y-CBT will help you change the way you respond to stress in your mind and body. It will help you develop a greater sense of well-being and boost your ability to handle stress with more resilience. These changes, in turn, will help you improve how you approach your relationships. You'll feel stronger and better able to face life's challenges with a new attitude—one marked by hope and an expectation of victory. Y-CBT can help you:

- Change the habits that keep you repeating the same anxious patterns over and over again

- Calm your racing thoughts

- Improve your body's reaction to stress so that you feel less physical anxiety in difficult situations

- Develop more positive feelings toward yourself

- Improve your communication with others

- Discover how to be guided by personal radiance rather than ruled by anxiety

Why We Created Y-CBT

We developed our unique six-week therapeutic Y-CBT program in response to a need that we identified while working at Riverside Community Care Outpatient Center, in Upton, Massachusetts. The center is one of many programs within Riverside Community Care's network of services. A nonprofit organization, Riverside provides children, adolescents, and adults with a broad range of behavioral health care and human services. Riverside programs provide services to more than forty thousand Massachusetts residents annually.

At Riverside's Upton center, we have met hundreds of people who lacked sufficient skills to manage symptoms of anxiety. Many believed that medication was their only tool. While medication can play an extremely valuable role in managing anxiety, we knew that there were other methods that could help too. We decided to offer people new skills to help pave the way for developing healthy life-long habits. As practitioners, we wanted to offer our clients a new path—a comprehensive approach that teaches people to have more control over the ways that symptoms of anxiety impact both their physical state and their thoughts.

Because anxiety has both physical and cognitive (thought) components, we sought to create a program that would address the *entire* experience of anxiety. We explored a combination of CBT, which targets the way we think (and subsequently behave), and the ancient practices of yoga and meditation, which have powerful calming effects on both our physical states and our thought processes.

And so we got started, creating a six-week group treatment model and piloting it in our practice. The results were dramatic and inspiring. Our clients reported that they were able to think more clearly when their bodies were calmer. They also found that when their minds were quieter, their bodies were less reactive to stress.

We conducted a research study (M. K. Khalsa et al. 2014) that confirmed that our clients were experiencing significant improvement. We concluded that the blend of these two established practices—CBT and yoga—resulted in a more complete resolution of our clients' anxiety. With these results, our group treatment program was established: Y-CBT Anxiety Management.

In writing this book, our goal is to share the methods of this promising new therapy with a much broader population. We hope that, by following the Y-CBT program set forth in these pages, you too will find relief from anxiety.

The self-help model presented here will benefit people who want to work on their own to address their anxiety issues. But we have also found that the model provides an effective adjunct for those who are working with a therapist and qualified prescriber to manage the more severe symptoms of anxiety. Additionally, this program can be beneficial in treating conditions that often co-occur, such as panic disorder and depression. Therapists who are seeking new strategies to help their clients deal with anxiety will also find this book useful, as will yoga students and teachers who have an interest in understanding anxiety from a therapeutic point of view.

It is very important to distinguish between the passing (and manageable) anxiety that most people feel and the more persistent, acute, problematic symptoms of anxiety that characterize an *anxiety disorder*.

Severe symptoms may require a psychiatric diagnosis and treatment. If you feel at any time that your symptoms are more than you can handle on your own, we recommend that you seek guidance and treatment from a behavioral health provider.

A licensed behavioral health provider will assess your symptoms and help you to access the right treatment for managing them. There are a number of anxiety disorders that people commonly struggle with today. In any twelve-month period, 18.1 percent of people in the United States experience the symptoms of an anxiety disorder (Kessler et al. 2005b). And 28.8 percent of us will experience the symptoms of this condition during the course of our lifetime (Kessler et al. 2005a). The *Diagnostic and Statistical Manual of Mental Disorders* (American Psychiatric Association 2013) lists several forms of anxiety disorders. Here some of the more common anxiety disorders:

Generalized anxiety disorder: characterized by excessive anxiety and worry lasting a long (at least six-month) period of time. The symptoms are very difficult to control and interfere with daily functioning.

Social anxiety disorder/social phobia: a specific fear that is centered on social interaction. It includes an intense, often debilitating fear leading to either avoiding social situations—including crowds and interactions with individuals—or enduring them with great distress.

Panic disorder: characterized by the regular occurrence of panic attacks, which include a sudden, explosive onset of frightening physical symptoms such as rapid heartbeat, an experience of choking, dizziness, and extreme fear, followed by the anticipatory anxiety that another attack will occur.

Agoraphobia: characterized by intense fear and anxiety related to being in open spaces, crowds, or using public transportation where escape might be difficult or embarrassing.

Regardless of the form anxiety takes, the symptoms can limit people's lives and potential. It is important that you give careful thought to the type of help that you need, be it using this book independently or seeking support from a qualified professional. Either way, we know that you can absolutely gain control over your symptoms of anxiety and lead a full and happy life.

When Science Meets Practice

For more than fifty years, therapists have been using cognitive behavioral therapy to help people suffering from anxiety. In 2008, Hofmann and Smits conducted a review of the available research and concluded that while CBT was effective, it could also benefit from improvement. In recent years, researchers have added techniques to enrich CBT with the hope of improving client outcomes. For example, in his groundbreaking work on stress reduction, Jon Kabat-Zinn added a mindfulness component to CBT with very good results (Segal, Williams, and Teasdale 2002).

During the last few decades, research has also supported the idea that yoga and meditation can reduce anxiety (Shannahoff-Khalsa 2004). In fact, many therapists have been using yoga, meditation, and breath training in their practices to treat anxiety—but without a formal, organized approach. Y-CBT provides such an approach by formally integrating these ancient practices with the modern techniques of CBT, resulting in a new and more effective method for managing anxiety.

Since 2008, the Riverside Community Care Outpatient Center has been the home of Y-CBT. Over the intervening years, we have used the techniques with groups and individuals in our practices. We have trained fellow therapists who now run Y-CBT groups in Riverside programs across the state.

Y-CBT has demonstrated excellent results. After the six-week program, people who participated in the Y-CBT groups showed significant reductions in anxiety and depression and also benefited from improved sleep (M. K. Khalsa et al. 2014). In a second study, the positive results have been substantiated, and we are continuing to conduct research on the effectiveness of the model (M. K. Khalsa, Greiner-Ferris, and Boisseau, forthcoming).

How to Use This Book

This book is based on the six-week Y-CBT Anxiety Management group treatment program that we have run in a clinic setting for several years. Participants meet once a week in a group and practice the techniques on their own the other six days. At the end of the program, we suggest that people continue a daily yoga and meditation practice, along with using Y-CBT techniques on a regular basis. The objective is to eventually embed these practices into their daily routine. This book is designed to be a do-it-yourself version of the six-week group treatment program that we offer our clients.

One Chapter a Week

We recommend that you read and work on one chapter a week, practicing the techniques as you go along. Be sure to follow the chapters in order, as each introduces new concepts that build on preceding material.

Each chapter consists of instruction and experience in *cognitive restructuring*, or learning to think differently, using principles of both CBT and yoga. You will also learn a variety of yoga and meditation techniques that can be both physically and emotionally calming.

In each program chapter you will find meditations and movements to learn and practice. These sets will help you better manage the physical symptoms of anxiety. You will also find worksheets and exercises that provide the opportunity to try out and reinforce the concepts as they are introduced. We have carefully selected and grouped the yoga, meditations, worksheets, and exercises. All together they form a comprehensive experience that will help you achieve the concepts set forth.

Most of the yoga and meditations are from the practices of Kundalini Yoga as taught by Yogi Bhajan®. These are marked with the letters KY. The yoga practice in this book is like a mini yoga class; please see the appendix to see the overall form of a Kundalini Yoga class. We have also included yoga, meditations, and exercises from other traditions, as well as some that we created ourselves.

Our overarching goal is to help you transform the way you manage your symptoms of stress and anxiety so they don't rule your existence or prevent you from living the life you want for yourself.

In the first chapter, "Understanding Yoga–Cognitive Behavioral Therapy," we present an overview of Y-CBT, the holistic benefits it confers, and the associated research. We also introduce the six Y-CBT guiding principles that will provide inspirational focal points and help you shift your core beliefs in a positive direction. In the second chapter, "The Mind-Body Connection," we explain current thinking on the mind-body connection and offer exercises and meditations to help you understand and experience this dynamic interplay. These first two chapters are foundational and provide background information to set the stage for the six-week program.

Week 1 of the program begins with the third chapter. Here we provide all of the tools necessary for starting a daily yoga and meditation practice. In Week 2, we dig deeper into anxiety and panic—how they affect your thoughts and your physical state. This is where you will really start to become aware of your own reactions to anxiety and begin to shift them into more calm and positive responses.

In Week 3, you will learn all about managing worry and how to change the thought patterns that are most common among those who struggle with anxiety.

Week 4 covers the importance of self-value and self-compassion, and teaches you how to increase these qualities within yourself. You'll learn how anxiety creates self-doubt and how the experience of fear can become life-limiting. Learning to recognize and embrace your intrinsic value will give you strength to face life's challenges. Week 5 deals with how anxiety can affect communication and relationships. You will learn how to hold on to your own value in difficult relationships and stressful communications. This chapter will help you understand your role in communication patterns and how to shift them to create a more positive interplay as you interact with others.

The final week of the program, Week 6, sets the foundation for you to continue a daily yoga and meditation practice, and use the Y-CBT program to fully uncover and nurture an inner strength that we call *personal radiance*. You will learn that when personal radiance is cultivated over time, you can use this tool to bring greater satisfaction to your life and interrupt patterns of anxiety. That is why the last chapter in our book is titled "Take Your Radiance out into the World." In it we leave you with words of encouragement and a wish for a radiant future.

We suggest that you alternate between reading about the ideas and practicing the related yoga and meditation. Creating this calmer state in your body will leave you more open to absorbing new ideas. Targeting the way that anxiety affects your mind and your body is central to the Y-CBT approach. Working on both simultaneously will help you transform your anxiety into a more complete state of calm in your mind, body, and even your spirit.

Together, the nine chapters in this book offer you comprehensive tools for developing a whole new way of approaching your life struggles. Over six weeks, you will build skills and learn concepts essential for creating a new daily practice and making real changes in your life.

Develop a New Practice

Your habits have been with you for a long time. Changing them will also take time—and *practice*. As you read this book, some ideas will be familiar to you, and some may be new. Some of the recommended techniques may be things you already believe could help but which you have been unable to incorporate into your life for one reason or another. This stumbling block captures one of the big frustrations in reading self-help books: sure, the idea may be good, but you just can't seem to carry it out or stick with it. Our program is different, because it helps you gradually build upon a daily practice that will enable you to make real and enduring changes.

You will develop your new routine by following the directions in the section called "Y-CBT Daily Practice," at the end of each week. Each of these practices builds on the preceding ones, helping you to create a daily routine that will become an essential part of achieving a quieter, calmer way of responding to stresses and challenges. Over time, your practice can help you move toward your full potential and attain the life goals you prize.

We know that developing a new routine is hard. Making changes means taking one step at a time. At first, you may want to use daily reminders, such as an alert on your mobile phone or a note on your calendar, to get you going each day. And *do* try to practice every day. The regularity will help you settle into your new routine. You will find that these daily sessions will help you face your day from a more centered and calm state. And when you do experience stress, you will begin to reflexively employ the skills that you have practiced. Expect that there will be days when you forget or are too tired to practice. When this happens, don't give up or be harsh with yourself. Every day, you have the opportunity to begin again. Over time, as you begin to see the effects of the work and the changes in yourself, you may naturally start to look forward to this peaceful time in your day.

A Y-CBT daily practice doesn't take much time—even five to ten minutes per day can be helpful. Nor does it require a trip to the gym, special workout clothes, or superior athletic ability. All it requires is your commitment to making your life, your mind, and your body quieter and more comfortable. If you set this goal for yourself, being consistent with your daily practice will come naturally.

The Y-CBT daily practice has four elements:

1. **A guiding principle:** A concept to contemplate for inspiration as you go through the week

2. **A yoga and meditation practice:** A time set aside daily to practice the yoga and meditation techniques taught in this book (Note: Yoga is always followed by meditation or relaxation.)

3. **A daily living practice:** The application of the techniques and activities offered in this book as you go about your day; the goal is to incorporate ways to help manage anxiety in your thoughts and your body whenever you have the need, day or night.

4. **A daily practice log:** A section at the end of every chapter where you can take notes and record your progress; we encourage you to use this tool, because committing thoughts to writing can have a powerful effect on memory and habit.

If you choose to read this book, we know you are looking for relief from anxiety. And we can help. In fact, we've already helped hundreds of people like you struggling with the same challenges. Many of our clients have made significant changes in their lives using the tools and techniques presented here. We have great confidence that *you too* can achieve these positive changes. Let's get started!

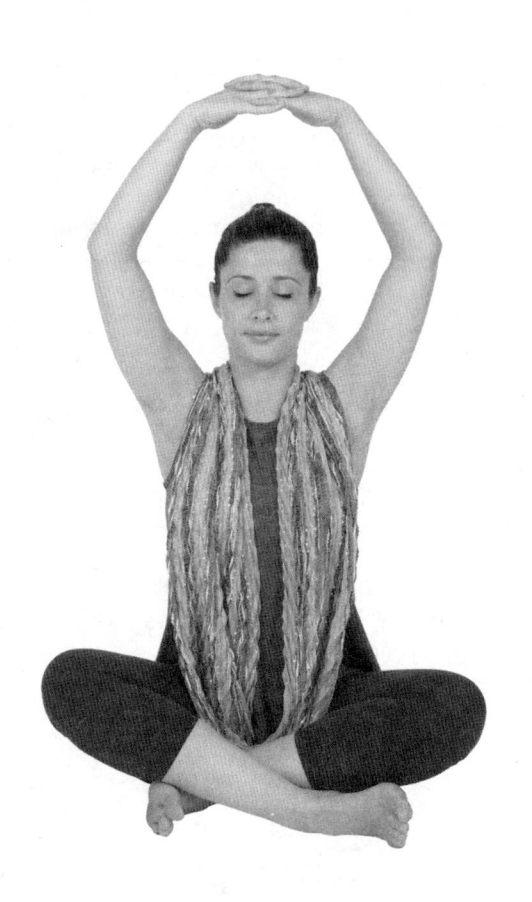

Understanding Yoga–Cognitive Behavioral Therapy

Aristotle said, "The whole is greater than the sum of its parts." His words held true for us as we created a new therapeutic approach to helping people who struggle with chronic anxiety and stress. Our integrative approach combines two effective treatments: cognitive behavioral therapy (CBT) and yoga and meditation (Y). Separately, each discipline has the power to help people overcome anxiety. Together, their effectiveness multiplies. Our blended approach, which we call Y-CBT, has helped many people manage anxiety and live a calmer, more fulfilling life. It can help you too.

Yoga and CBT are natural partners, with many commonalities. Both of them:

- Acknowledge that patterns of thought influence our emotional states, and that changing the workings of the mind can help us resolve emotional turmoil

- Help us shift our outlook when we get stuck in negative thought patterns, so that we can see other possibilities

- Operate on the belief that we are able to control our thoughts and the activity of our minds

- Encourage a simple, forthright focus on the *present moment* that is central to achieving an improved state of being

Neither yoga nor CBT will solve all facets of your struggle with emotional distress. Yoga alone does not fully address the content of thought, and CBT alone does not fully target the physical discomfort that so commonly accompanies emotional distress.

When yoga and cognitive behavioral therapy are blended together, the whole becomes greater than the sum of its parts.

Cognitive Behavioral Therapy

Cognitive behavioral therapy as a formal theory evolved from the work of psychiatrist Aaron Beck and psychologist Albert Ellis in the 1950s and '60s. The primary tenet of CBT is that negative and faulty patterns of thinking affect a person's emotional state and behavior. The goal of CBT is to help people *rework the way they think*, thus changing problematic thought patterns to more productive ones. These changes, in turn, can improve the way people feel and also change patterns of behavior.

CBT teaches people to identify their unique negative thought processes and core beliefs, and to gradually begin to shift these cognitive activities to more accurate and constructive patterns of thinking. The ultimate goal is to develop a more positive outlook on life's challenges.

For example, a person who is anxious may have the generalized belief "I'm going to fail." In CBT sessions, the therapist helps the person understand the source of this faulty belief, challenge its validity, and amend the limiting belief to a more productive and useful concept, such as "There are steps that I can take to become successful in my life."

A distressed person may hold on to destructive thoughts and beliefs with great conviction. With help, an anxious person can learn to view negative beliefs as hypotheses rather than facts and to test them out by running "experiments" that try out new ways of thinking and behaving.

When undergoing cognitive behavioral therapy, people are also encouraged to monitor and log the *automatic thoughts* that pop into their minds. This task helps identify the underlying patterns and allows for the development of more adaptive alternatives. CBT is a problem-focused approach to therapy, often using worksheets and weekly homework.

How Effective Is CBT?

CBT is often considered the gold standard for the treatment of anxiety, and more than two hundred research articles have affirmed its efficacy in reducing anxiety (Knaus 2014). A 2007 review of the literature found that CBT demonstrated strong positive outcomes in treating panic disorder, agoraphobia, social anxiety disorder, obsessive-compulsive disorder (OCD), and generalized anxiety disorder as well as post-traumatic stress disorder (Norton and Price 2007). CBT research has also begun to consider the role of physiological factors in anxiety (Borkovec et al. 2002), and relaxation techniques can also serve as an important component of a CBT program (Knaus 2014).

While CBT is often very effective, treatment outcomes may be enhanced with the addition of other techniques. Some people who try this therapy continue to experience some degree of anxiety, and others don't respond as well as we might like (Evans et al. 2008). Our goal in developing Y-CBT is to integrate the most successful aspects of CBT with the power of yoga, in an effort to treat anxiety more completely. While CBT can help alter our negative thinking, yoga is particularly effective at addressing the physical discomfort of emotional distress.

Yoga

Yoga is said to have begun thousands of years ago in ancient India (Feuerstein 2008). It was originally an oral tradition, a practice passed from teacher to student, and the first texts on the subject didn't appear until about 2,000 years ago.

The practice of yoga involves an extensive system of exercise that engages both the mind (cognitive and meditative concentration) and the body (postures and breathing exercises), and can promote feelings of well-being, both physically and emotionally.

Our bodies are programmed biochemically to react to stimuli such as stress, criticism, noise, unfamiliar situations, or bad news in certain ways that are not always positive or healthy. Yoga can help reduce these automatic anxious responses to the everyday circumstances of our lives. We may have learned to be emotionally reactive, or we may have been born with the tendency, but in either case yoga can help the body respond to stress and other events more calmly and with less reactivity.

Yoga is also beneficial to the mind. The regular practice of yoga is said to have a positive impact on the nervous and glandular systems. Balancing and improving these systems enhances brain function, which leads to calmer, more focused thinking. Studies have demonstrated that practicing yoga can significantly reduce anxiety (S. B. Khalsa and Cope 2006; Kirkwood et al. 2005) and enhance mood (Streeter et al. 2010). It can also help to reduce depression (Shapiro et al. 2007), sleep disturbance, hypertension, and headaches (Field 2011). One literature review of 150 studies revealed that yoga significantly reduced anxiety in patients with a variety of medical conditions (S. B. S. Khalsa 2004).

Meditation

Meditation is also believed to have started thousands of years ago in India (Feuerstein 2008). The word "meditation" is widely used today to describe an extensive array of contemplative practices, most of which have the common goal of controlling one's attention. Today, people meditate to relax, to improve their mood, and to enhance their overall sense of well-being in body and mind.

Our nervous systems often react to difficult situations using familiar, repetitive pathways that can lead to anxiety. One form of meditation, called *mindfulness*, has received increasing attention from scientists who study the brain. Research shows that meditation appears to change the way the brain processes emotional situations, in effect short-circuiting these familiar pathways so that the body naturally relaxes, even in the face of difficulties (Gard et al. 2014).

After meditating, people report improved mood and lower levels of anxiety and reactivity (Gard et al. 2014; Lutz et al. 2008). *Self-compassion*, or the kindness you feel toward yourself, also improves with meditation (Neff 2003). This lessening of negative feelings about yourself represents an important step toward enhanced mental health. With the consistent practice of meditation, the mind becomes calmer and people experience less depression and anxiety (Neff, Kirkpatrick, and Rude 2007).

Yoga is often considered a kind of "meditation in motion" (S. B. Khalsa et al. 2009). In our work, we use yoga and meditations from the traditions of Kundalini Yoga.

Kundalini Yoga and Meditation

There are many styles of yoga and meditation, all which have documented beneficial effects. Kundalini Yoga (KY) is known as the yoga of awareness, and its goal is to help you achieve your *highest potential*, growing into the person you truly want to be.

Kundalini Yoga and meditation incorporate many of the ancient yoga poses. It also emphasizes breathing, exercises, and chanting. The word "kundalini" refers to the sacred energy that is said to reside at the base of the spine, and this method of yoga was traditionally designed to access that energy. Yogi Bhajan, who lived from 1929 to 2004, learned yoga as a child in India from one of the masters. He is credited with bringing Kundalini Yoga to the West in the late 1960s.

The sequences of KY yoga postures and the meditations in this book are said to reduce anxiety, strengthen the nervous and glandular systems, and produce a relaxing and invigorating impact on mind and body. When practiced every day, KY can be very effective at calming the mind and reducing anxiety and depression.

In two controlled studies, Kundalini Yoga was shown to significantly reduce the anxiety associated with OCD (Shannahoff-Khalsa 2004) and to improve cognitive functioning in older people (Watts 2016). Other studies have shown that KY can benefit the heart (Peng et al. 1999) and decrease anxiety and stress in those suffering from PTSD (Jindani, Turner, and Khalsa 2015).

Yoga–Cognitive Behavioral Therapy

Y-CBT is an evolution of contemporary psychological thought and practice related to anxiety. In order to experience complete relief from worry and anxiety, you need to work on making changes in both your physical *and* cognitive responses to stress. By blending the cognitive benefits of CBT with the physical and psychological benefits of yoga, Y-CBT targets the way you think and feel as well as your metabolic systems. We have found that this combination leads to a faster and more integrated resolution of symptoms.

For several years, we have conducted research at the Riverside Community Care Outpatient Center, in Upton, Massachusetts. In a recently published study, we looked at the effectiveness of Y-CBT for people who were experiencing severe anxiety (many also suffered from depression and other psychological issues). After the six-week Y-CBT treatment, people's *state anxiety* (that is, anxiety *felt in the moment*) dropped by 23 percent, while their *trait anxiety* (the *tendency to react* with anxiety) fell by 16 percent. In addition, their depression was reduced by 47 percent (M. K. Khalsa et al. 2014).

Y-CBT is a progressive journey. As you read through the chapters and practice the exercises, you will develop a deepening sense of self-awareness and internal growth. This expanded experience of self is empowering and can transform many facets of your life, including how you work with your anxiety, your sadness, your self-esteem, and even your relationships.

As the Y-CBT process lowers your anxiety and lifts your sadness, it also builds a more positive experience of yourself and a greater sense of well-being. You will also find a change in the way you interact with the people you care about. This is because an anxious state often keeps you inwardly focused, guarded, and disconnected from others. By reducing the discomfort that comes with anxiety, Y-CBT techniques can help diminish this inward focus. Consequently, you may find that you are able to interact with others in a warmer, more authentic manner.

Y-CBT Techniques

Y-CBT incorporates a range of techniques to restructure the negative patterns of anxiety, both physical and psychological. One such technique, which you will learn about in Week 3, is the Victory

Meditation. In this exercise, you combine a physical state (by raising your arm in the air and doing controlled, segmented breathing) with a specific thought (concentrating on the word and meaning of *victory*). This pairing is very effective in calming both the mind and the body.

Learning to take control of your thoughts is central to reducing the process of worry and rumination, and cognitive behavioral therapy teaches you to replace the content of a negative thought with a new thought. Restructuring your thoughts in this way has been shown to reduce distorted thinking and therefore reduce anxiety. Y-CBT combines techniques such as this with ideas based on yoga and meditation to help you learn to shift your thought process. Physical movements, spinal postures, and breath exercises hold equal importance in helping achieve an overall calmer state. Y-CBT also encourages you to allow, observe, and let go of problematic thoughts as they arise, and it offers wisdom and self-compassion as keys to allowing alternative ways of thinking.

Engaging these mental and physical responses to anxiety and stress activates different parts of the brain and allows you to deactivate the brain's "default" response, thereby reducing the rumination that can lead to anxiety.

In combination with these techniques, Y-CBT rests on a set of core principles that offer a framework for the process of change.

Y-CBT Guiding Principles

The theory and practices of Y-CBT revolve around a set of six principles that will steer your journey toward positive change. These guiding principles act as touchstones as you learn Y-CBT and progress through the program presented in this book. They will help you reconceptualize your negative or self-defeating beliefs and replace them with alternative healing concepts.

Each week of the program has at its core a different guiding principle. We encourage you to consider incorporating these ideas into the core beliefs that guide *your* life as well. Each week, be sure to devote some time to contemplating the associated guiding principle and what it means to you.

Everyone is capable of great courage and has a remarkable ability to change. All of us can create a calm place from which we can face our thoughts, emotions, and relationships.

The mind and body are fluidly connected. The state of the mind is dependent on the state of the body, and vice versa. As one shifts, the other will follow in kind.

Relief can be found in facts. Freedom from worry and anxiety can often be found by focusing on the facts or objective truth of the situation rather than on a fragmented understanding or fantasy-driven fear.

Habits of the mind influence our lives. What we think affects how we feel. Our thoughts are of our own making. As we are the only ones who are thinking our thoughts, we can choose to create habits of mind that give us peace and success.

There is a "reciprocal loop" in all communication. In every encounter between individuals, there is a back-and-forth interaction that creates the mood and the message between the participants. Awareness and ownership of how we influence our interactions is profoundly important in the development of healthy and satisfying relationships.

Our intentions help to focus our attention. The simple act of attending to ourselves—our body, our breath, our thoughts—with nurturing acceptance and encouragement is a powerful mechanism for change. It is important that we come to understand the goals that underlie our thoughts, words, and actions. These are not always conscious, and they are critical.

Common Questions About Yoga and Meditation

If yoga and meditation are new to you, you may have a lot of questions. It may feel strange or even intimidating to try the techniques we offer in the following chapters. Many people feel this way at first but become more comfortable as they experience the benefits over time. Here are some of the most common questions our clients and students ask.

How hard is the yoga in this program?

The yoga and meditations we have selected are simple and can be done by almost everyone. The goal is for you to gain benefit from the yoga. You don't need to do the poses *perfectly* to begin to feel the effects. You should be mindful of any injuries or medical conditions you have and adapt or simplify the movements based on your particular needs. It you have an injury or experience any pain or discomfort with a particular movement, simply sit quietly and imagine in your mind's eye that you are completing the movement. What's important is that you are focusing on the movements, correcting your breath, and doing the best you can.

What is the pace of the yoga in this program?

The pace of Kundalini Yoga follows the rhythm of the breath. The movement between poses is smooth and fluid. Popular forms of yoga you may have seen on TV often use large, dynamic, and sometimes intricate movements that start from standing and go to the floor and back up again. While Kundalini Yoga also uses these poses, in addition it incorporates small, sometimes rapid movements concentrated on just one or two muscle groups that affect particular systems of the body (such as the heart or nervous system). The yoga that we have chosen for this program is designed to be accessible to most everyone—it's low impact, nonstrenuous, and easy on the joints. For this book, we use poses that can be practiced in a seated position, either on the floor or in a chair.

How do I breathe correctly?

In general, anxious breathing has several elements: it is shallow and fast and often involves exhaling through the mouth. The healthy way is to use Natural Breathing (see Week 2), a very simple but effective and calming breath. This breath is done from the diaphragm and through the nose, with about five inhales and exhales per minute. In the yoga and meditation instructions, specific breathing patterns are usually specified. Most breathing is done through the nose, unless a specific mouth breath is described. We encourage you to resist any impulse you may have to breathe through your mouth, unless the set calls for it.

Do I need to have experience?

No. Beginners and experienced practitioners alike will find it relatively easy to follow the directions and the pictures in the following chapters, and enjoy the benefits of these meditations and exercises. If you are a beginner, start by practicing the exercises for just one minute each; a more experienced person may practice longer and thereby have a deeper experience.

In Summary

Although it is a relatively new method, Y-CBT has shown great promise in helping people manage anxiety. Many of our clients report that their ability to calm themselves has dramatically improved, that they feel less depressed, and that they have an increased ability to solve their problems with greater clarity. Fellow clinicians who use Y-CBT in their practices have echoed these results. The combination of the physical movements and philosophies of yoga, along with the behavioral interventions of CBT, shows great promise as a treatment for the symptoms of anxiety.

We are thrilled to have you participate in this program. It may feel as if your freedom from overwhelming anxiety will never come. But we believe that if you make it to the end of this book and have incorporated the yoga, writing exercises, and meditations we teach into a daily practice, you *will* see results in six weeks—even sooner in many cases.

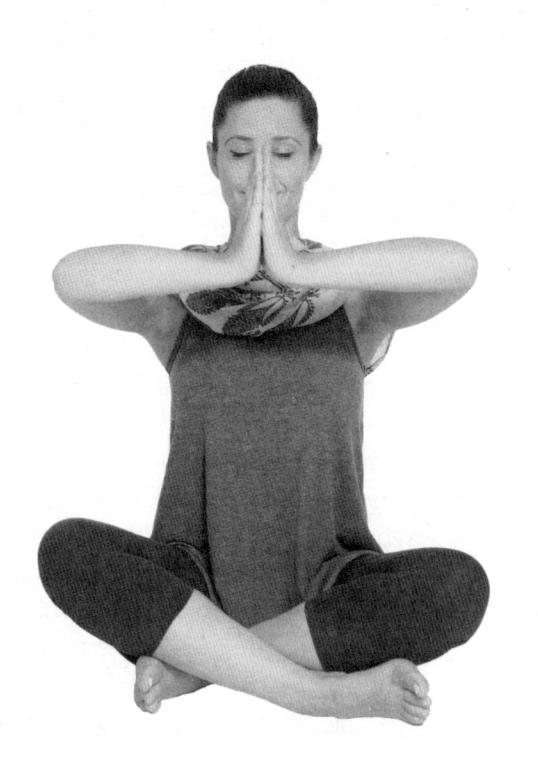

The Mind-Body Connection

I n this chapter, we explore the connection between your mind and your body, and how profoundly anxiety affects both. You will learn how to address and reduce the intense physical discomfort of stress and anxiety, and how to create a sense of calm and comfort in your body.

Understanding the relationship between your anxious thoughts and your physical responses to stress is central to reducing your overall level of anxiety. It is impossible to simply "think your way out" of a problem. The ping-pong between cognition and the physiologic effects of stress creates a cycle that you need to resolve in order to build a lasting sense of strength-based calm to face the unpredictable challenges life places in your path.

The Nature of the Mind

People have been philosophizing about the nature of mind for centuries. One of the most authoritative texts on yoga, Patanjali's *Yoga Sutras*, was written some two thousand years ago and is still used today. This collection of *sutras*, or aphorisms, focuses on the qualities of the mind and how to relate to them in order to reduce suffering (Feuerstein 2008).

The mind is multilayered and complex, and it can be your dear friend or a terrible enemy (Bhajan and Khalsa 1998), so it's important to understand its nature. We can characterize the mind as an automatic mechanism that processes sensations and thoughts. While it can at times be quiet and calm, it's often very "noisy," releasing thousands of thoughts and images in rapid succession, some of which are helpful while others are self-critical and harmful. Your own mind can generate a solution for you then turn on you with unrelenting criticism if that solution fails (Bhajan and Khalsa 1998).

The mind is constantly judging things in order to assess options; it generates and compares pros and cons, positives and negatives. Often, the mind will produce both positive and negative thoughts on the same topic (Bhajan 2003). For example, it's common to feel both love and anger toward someone you love. This dichotomy can be confusing!

Your mind is in endless motion, and it is easily influenced by external factors, such as food and conversation, and by physiological factors, such as your biochemistry and breathing patterns. It can shift in response to people and circumstances, and even to its own thoughts.

Storytelling is central to the human experience, and the mind is a master storyteller. It constructs stories that can be filled with inaccurate interpretations of reality. These distorted stories cloud the mind, as though cloaking it in a filmy color (Bhajan and Khalsa 1998; Desikachar 1995). But the mind continues to narrate, often repeating the same stories over and over.

How you respond to this narration determines whether the voice in your head guides you well or works against you. It's all too easy to get caught in the tangled web of the mind, so it's important to create habits of mind that foster confidence, success, and happiness. You can learn to attend to the process of how you communicate within yourself and ultimately rise above the unruly nature of the mind to find a *neutral mind*. This book will teach you how to use meditation, mindfulness, and yoga to find a stable point of stillness from which to observe and befriend the mind so that it becomes your ally (Bajan 2003). But first, let's look at the mind's home: the body.

Your Body Is Your Home

The body—your physical self—is the place where your mind resides. Your body is the place where your emotions, thoughts, and beliefs are contained. Your body is therefore the home to all that you are.

Physical symptoms of anxiety can make your body feel like a hostile environment that you long to escape from. Indeed, most people who struggle with anxiety can relate to the urge to "disconnect" from the body. The phrase "I was climbing out of my skin" aptly describes the feeling. Without the skills to manage these symptoms, people often engage in behaviors that may prolong the problem, or, in the long run, make their situations worse. For instance, some people will begin to avoid all situations that make them anxious, and their lives then become very limited. Can you relate to this?

Learning to become aware of, consciously connected to, and in control of the condition of your bodily home is essential if you hope to achieve and maintain an overall state of tranquility and strength as you face life's inevitable challenges.

Your mind and your body are fully entwined and have a powerful, fluid effect on one another. The mind and the body respond simultaneously to all of your experiences. When facing stress or fear, your reaction is an interwoven cognitive and physiologic process.

You can quiet your mind by relaxing your body, and you can quiet the discomfort of your body by quieting your mind.

Anxious thoughts, worry, and rumination have the power to trap you in your mind. Indeed, these states of emotion and thought are profoundly engaging. When lost in an anxious thought process, *thinking* is all that you can think about. This all-consuming process creates a disconnect from what is going on within your own body. To remedy that disconnect, you need to create a comfortable home.

Building a Comfortable Home

Creating this relaxed and comfortable physical home is within your power. First, you have to nurture yourself. For optimal mental and physical health, your body needs daily attention and care: healthy food, quality sleep, positive social interaction, and lots of exercise.

But instead of providing yourself with this nourishment, you might often push yourself to the limit and get overwhelmed by work, family responsibilities, and other demands. Are we right? Attending to the state of the physical self is pivotal in the process of managing stress and anxiety.

Below is a list of common expressions that people use to describe how anxiety makes their bodies feel. If you answer yes to any of the following questions, then you have a good idea of what anxiety feels like in the body.

Have you described your body as "a bundle of nerves"?

Have you ever discovered after a day of worry and distress that your body feels like you have been in a boxing match?

After a period of high stress, does your head throb?

Do your legs ever feel wobbly?

Do certain situations literally *take your breath away*?

These and other feelings and symptoms arise from the profound physical changes that take place in the body when you experience anxiety. These effects can range from general musculoskeletal discomfort to chronic health issues (Hoffman, Dukes, and Wittchen 2008).

Learning how to actively attend to and respond to your physical self in the face of stressful situations will help you create a comfortable home from which you can effectively face the stresses of life. Becoming aware of your unique physical reactions to stress is the first step in taming them. The following exercise will launch you on this discovery process.

EXERCISE:
Your Physical Reaction to Stress

Becoming aware of your stress responses is the first step to creating a safe, comfortable bodily home. What are the physical symptoms that you experience when you are under stress? What are the sensations that make your body feel like a hostile environment?

Check all that apply:

_____ Tension in the back and neck

_____ Racing heart or palpitations

_____ Nausea or stomachaches

_____ Overall internal agitation

_____ Tightness in the chest

_____ Shaking hands, arms, or legs

_____ Headaches

_____ Chronic restlessness

_____ Other: _____

Automatic Behavioral Responses

In addition to these physical reactions, we all develop automatic, reflexive *behavioral responses* to unpleasant or stressful experiences. These knee-jerk reactions happen because, when something feels uncomfortable, our natural reflex is to *do something* to make it stop. People who have struggled with symptoms of anxiety often develop problematic or self-defeating responses.

EXERCISE:
Your Automatic Behavioral Response to Stress

What automatic habits have you acquired in response to anxiety? Below is a list of common self-defeating or unhealthy behaviors that many people develop. Check any that apply to you:

_____ Run, retreat, or hide

_____ Fight, argue, or attack

_____ Get high, drink, or take a pill

_____ Eat

_____ Other: _____

Creating a New Automatic Physical Reflex

Believe it or not, your physical *and* behavioral responses to stressful events *are within your control.* At first, this may sound like a startling concept, especially if your responses, such as muscle tension when stressed or bingeing on junk food when anxious, seem automatic and feel as though they are outside of your ability to choose. It may even feel as if a force outside of yourself controls your physical state.

But once you begin to understand your habits and your physical responses to stress, you can start to replace negative behaviors with healthier, more productive ones. Instead of becoming tense and reactive at the first sign of stress, you can learn to respond calmly by breathing mindfully, relaxing your muscles, and dropping your shoulders.

The following exercise will teach you to develop a new automatic physical reflex, one that involves breathing and relaxing your muscles. As you become practiced and proficient in taking charge and shifting your response, you will find yourself reacting differently to the real-life stressful moments that occur, creating a comfortable home for your mind instead.

EXERCISE:
Change Your Automatic Reaction to Stress

Changing your automatic behavioral responses is the next step in taking control of your physical self and creating a safe, comfortable physical home. The goal of this exercise is to learn how to relax your body and your mind when you are feeling stressed rather than automatically tensing up, which will ultimately lead to negative, distressing thoughts.

1. First, list several stress-inducing situations that produce a physical response in you. List them in order of the level of anxiety you feel, from low (1) to high (4).

   _____

   _____

   _____

   _____

2. Pick the situation that causes the lowest level of anxiety for you (later you can practice with the more challenging situations).

3. Next, sit quietly in a comfortable place. Visualize the stressful situation with as much detail as you can. Take your time to picture in your mind's eye the events, the details, the conversation, and so forth. Allow the stress-induced physical sensations to occur. Observe and take note of where they occur in your body.

4. Now, respond to the physical reaction to the stress by relaxing and calming those areas of your body. Keep your eyes closed. Drop your shoulders. Take a long deep breath. Exhale fully. Repeat.

Practice these steps a little bit every day. It takes time to unlearn the responses to stress that you have developed over time, but you *can* develop a new automatic response.

The important thing to remember is to take a deep breath and relax your body and your mind when you are feeling stressed. As you become comfortable with this exercise, you can use it to visualize more stressful situations. Over time, you will notice that your automatic tensing responses are waning, with relaxed and calming responses taking their place.

Mindfulness

Mindfulness is used in psychotherapy today to reach a quiet, nonjudgmental state of mind from which one can calmly observe unwanted thoughts. Jon Kabat Zinn introduced this concept to the world of traditional psychology in the 1970's. As a practitioner of Buddhist meditation, he was able to effectively integrate meditation with traditional cognitive behavioral therapy. Kabat Zinn called this new method Mindfulness-Based-Stress-Reduction (MSBR). The model was very successful, and he established the Stress Reduction Clinic and The Center for Mindfulness at the University of Massachusetts Medical Center, where he still serves as Professor of Medicine Emeritus. Backed by a large number of studies (Hofmann, Sawyer, Witt & Oh, 2010; De Bruin, van der Zwan & Bogels, 2016) mindfulness has become very popular in psychology and has helped many people to feel less depressed and less anxious.

The practice of mindfulness asks us to be fully present in the moment—aware of all the sensations around us, allowing problematic thoughts to pass by without focusing on them (Segal, Williams, and Teasdale 2002). People often try to ignore or push away upsetting, anxious thoughts, countering with mental pleas such as *Go away! I don't want to think about this anymore* or *Oh, No! I shouldn't feel this way—I have to stop!*

But attempting to suppress a thought may actually strengthen it. Pushing it away gives it attention, which makes it stronger. It's as if, when pushed away, the thought pushes back, forcing you to muster further energy to resist it. This process is tiring and can cloud your thinking, which can, in turn, result in more anxiety and self-criticism.

Think of the game tug-of-war, in which two teams pull on opposite ends of a rope, creating a great tension. When you fight with your own thoughts, the push and pull that anxious thinking sets off can be all-consuming. When you engage a mindful posture, you in effect "drop the rope." Letting go of a thought, rather than fighting it, reduces the tension you feel and opens up the possibility of calm.

The ability to approach life's challenges from an objective and nonjudgmental perspective is not easy, but it is well worth striving to attain. Instead of trying to *stop* yourself from thinking about something or to *change* your thoughts about it, you can learn to *accept* what you are thinking and *allow* those thoughts to occur. Ultimately, this new way of relating to your thoughts will increase your ability to tolerate anxiety and strong emotions.

Now let's try it out. The next two guided meditations will give you practice in observing thoughts and sensations using mindfulness.

MEDITATION:
Observing Thoughts

This meditation will help you learn how to observe your thoughts. It gives you the opportunity to simply observe the state of your mind.

1. Sit quietly and comfortably. Close your eyes.

2. Take a few deep breaths to center yourself.

3. Listen to the thoughts that begin to emerge in your mind.

4. Attend to the thoughts as if you are watching a movie or listening to the radio.

5. Listen as though you can't engage or change the thoughts.

6. Simply observe.

7. Continue this for up to 1 minute.

8. Take a deep breath and relax. Open your eyes.

MEDITATION:
Observing Sensations

This meditation will help you to become aware of the sensations that you are experiencing at this moment. It offers you the opportunity to simply observe your physical state.

1. Sit quietly and comfortably. Close your eyes.

2. Take a few deep breaths to center yourself.

3. Place your hand palm-side down on a smooth surface such as a wall, a tabletop, or a book.

4. Note the temperature of the smooth surface.

5. Keep your hand in that place, and focus only on the temperature for 5 seconds.

6. Take the temperature of a second surface in the same way.

7. Focus only on the temperature for 5 seconds.

8. Take a deep breath and relax. Open your eyes.

These two guided meditations can help sharpen your ability to observe what is happening in your mind and body, and increase your awareness of the richness of the present moment. These meditations can be practiced anytime and in any posture or location. They can be especially helpful when your mind is racing from one anxious thought to another. Taking these moments to just *be, sit,* and *observe* can often help to break the racing thought and allow for a calmer mind. We think you'll find that these techniques are more effective than trying to think your way out of a problem, as you will see in the next section.

Why We Can't Think Our Way out of a Problem

The mind is very tricky, as you've discovered—it creates intrigue and is constantly going back and forth between the positive and the negative. For this reason, it can be very difficult to "think" your way out of a problem.

During the past thirty years, MRI studies have identified a neural network in the brain that people use when their attention is not focused and occupied. The network has been aptly called the *default mode network* (DMN) because it is the neural pathway that the brain recruits by default when attention is not engaged (Broyd et al. 2009).

Simple passive tasks or "resting" activities such as watching television, daydreaming, and even driving a car on automatic pilot can engage the DMN. This neural network is associated with depression, rumination, and anxiety. It is difficult to escape these emotions while the DMN is active, but engaging other neural pathways may be an effective way to become less depressed, ruminative, or anxious (Hasenkamp et al. 2012). Controlling your attention through active tasks such as working on a computer or doing mindfulness exercises can serve to engage other areas of the brain to bring you out of the default mode network.

Brain-imaging studies have confirmed that meditation and mindfulness may reduce the rumination and mind wandering associated with the DMN (Hasenkamp et al. 2012). Other evidence suggests that long-term meditators can deactivate parts of the DMN to a greater degree than beginner meditators can. This deactivation is associated with reduced emotional intensity (Taylor et al. 2011), and it may also lead to more-positive interpretations of events. Mindfulness may even reduce the number of negative thoughts that arise in the first place (Lutz et al. 2008).

In Summary

Understanding the mind-body connection and the relationship between your thoughts and your physical response to stress is key to reducing your overall level of anxiety. The first steps are to become aware of your automatic responses, and then to begin to take charge of and shift your reactions. Observing your thoughts and sensations will help you really get to know yourself and what happens to you when under stress. You have learned some of the basics in this chapter, and it may be helpful to review it from time to time as you move through the book.

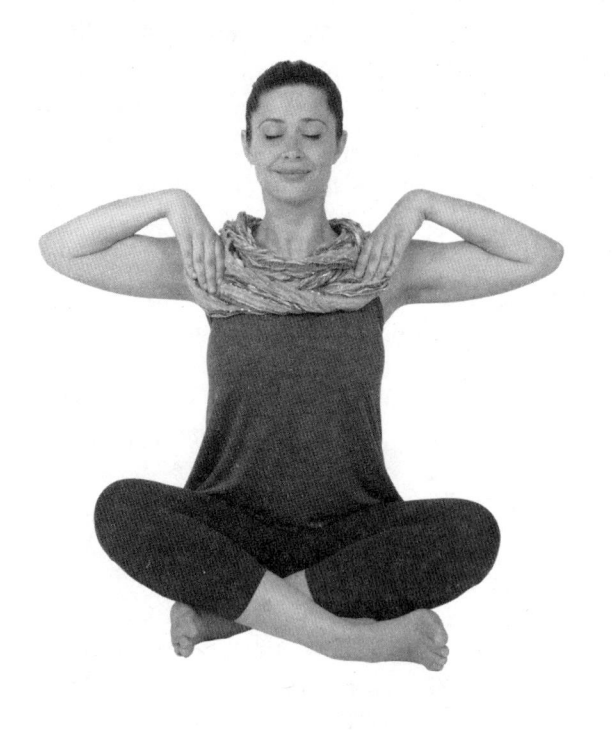

WEEK 1

Establishing a Daily Practice

Anxiety is a frightening experience. For some people, the experience is so uncomfortable that they make adjustments to their daily routines to avoid these terrible, uncomfortable feelings. Many people avoid certain situations, interactions, or relationships as a means to protect themselves from the overwhelming discomfort. This is how anxiety becomes life-limiting.

Changing your response to anxiety by learning a *new* way of responding takes courage. Simply by picking up this book and resolving to make changes, you have taken a brave and vital step. In this chapter, which presents Week 1 of our six-week program, we explain the importance of developing a daily practice to help you in this process of change. A daily yoga and meditation practice is one of the most effective ways to develop what we call *attention in action*. This term describes a state of being that makes use of self-compassion, intention, and self-control so that what you pay attention to is under your control and your focus serves to reduce your anxiety.

As you begin, consider this week's Y-CBT guiding principle: ***Everyone is capable of great courage and has a remarkable ability to change.***

As you may well know, anxiety can cause people to retreat from their lives in an effort to feel safe from stress and conflict. Finding the courage within yourself to begin to make changes will ultimately lead to a fuller life, because you will no longer feel the need to hide from certain situations and people. Remember, courage doesn't mean having no fears; it means that you have resolved to move forward in spite of them. Use this week's guiding principle as an affirmation to remind yourself that you *can* make changes.

The Y-CBT Daily Practice

All of us develop habits and certain behaviors over time. So it should come as no surprise that it will take time and discipline to change these entrenched patterns. Instructors of yoga or meditation will often use the phrase "developing a practice." That's because those who follow these Eastern traditions believe that a regular daily practice is key to achieving a more aware, relaxed state of being that is sustainable over a lifetime. The challenge, then, is to set aside a time every day for your practice. With consistency, this practice will become an essential part of your life.

The Y-CBT daily practice has four parts: the guiding principle of the week, the yoga and meditation set, the daily living practice, and the practice log. Each chapter also includes additional exercise recommendations for your practice that week.

While there are common elements to the condition we call anxiety, each person responds somewhat differently to different triggers. Each week you will learn new concepts, strategies, and techniques to help you focus on a particular aspect of how anxiety affects *you*. Using these tools, you will learn to pay very close attention to the complex elements of your own thoughts and the emotional and physical manifestations of anxiety. You will then practice techniques that target these reactions and that promote more helpful, soothing, and compassionate ways of responding. Some of the Y-CBT strategies are meant to be used as you go about your day, while others are meant to be included in your formal daily practice.

Your Y-CBT Daily Practice

Develop a routine to complete the four steps of the daily practice. Each day:

1. Review the guiding principle.
2. Do the yoga and meditation set.
3. Integrate the daily living practice suggestions.
4. Fill out the practice log.

Elements of a Yoga and Meditation Practice

Choose a regular time of day for your daily practice. We recommend a morning practice, because it can help set a calm and peaceful rhythm for your day. The amount of time needed will vary from week to week, depending on the work assigned. This week's practice should take five to ten minutes per day.

In yogic terms, a daily practice is called *sadhana*, which is a quiet time for nourishing yourself emotionally, physically, and spiritually (S. P. K. Khalsa 2007). In a way, a daily practice is like a soothing warm bath—it cleans away the emotional debris that clogs your mind and body. It is a time to respect and care for your body and your mind, always recognizing that the state of one will follow the other. This nurturing *sadhana* will help put you in a serene state so that you can be more patient, kind, and compassionate with yourself and others.

Before You Start

First, be sure you are comfortable. Try not to eat more than a light snack up to an hour or so before you begin. Wear loose-fitting, natural-fiber clothing that allows you to move easily. Have some fresh water on hand and a cushion to sit on, if you like.

Find a quiet place. Any spot will do, but if possible choose a beautiful, quiet area, perhaps with an array of candles or another pleasant focal point. This is a time to pay complete attention to yourself. It is best to turn off electronic devices and shut out unwanted sounds, if possible. Of course, in some households, especially those with children, complete silence may not always be feasible. That's not a problem—learning to tolerate ambient sounds can be worked into the meditations.

During Your Practice

Consciously relax your body. Breathe deeply. Become aware of your sensations. Notice the way your skin feels; listen to the sounds around you.

Consciously become aware of the content of your thoughts and simply observe them without judgment. With your eyes closed, focus your mind at the point between your eyebrows. You may simply focus there, or you may picture a neutral image of something, perhaps a smooth stone. Try to let go of tensions.

Be sure to carefully follow the instructions for each yoga set, particularly with regard to time and duration. These sets are like recipes; if, for example, you lengthen the time of one movement, be sure to lengthen the rest of the set proportionally. Also, be sure to do the exercises in the order given, as they are designed to work in a systematic way to achieve the desired results.

Always end your practice time with a period of relaxation or meditation. This is important for two reasons: First, a period of quiet breathing and relaxation after the exercises will enhance the effects of the yoga. Second, the practice of yoga focuses your attention and helps to balance your nervous and glandular systems, thus calming your mind and body so that you are better prepared to meditate.

Rating Your Progress

It is helpful to keep track of your progress and the techniques you're using. Use the table at the end of each chapter to do this. Make note of the exercises and techniques that work well for you so that you can revisit and practice them after you complete the six-week program.

Using a scale of 1 to 10, rate your anxiety *before* you try the technique. Practice the technique, and then rate your anxiety *after* you finish. Once you begin to experience some relief from anxiety, it can be easy to forget how far you've come. You can look back on your practice logs regularly to remind yourself of how much progress you've made.

Important Tips for Your Yoga and Meditation Practice

Here are some ways to get the most benefit from your daily practice:

- Practice the yoga exercises in the order given.

- Maintain the timing ratios. It's okay to do shorter sessions, just be sure to change the timing of all of the exercises proportionally.

- Always follow yoga with a period of meditation or relaxation.

More Questions About Yoga and Meditation

We answered some of the most common initial questions in the first chapter, "Understanding Yoga–Cognitive Behavioral Therapy." Here are some more.

What is Easy Pose?

The meditations and most of the exercises in this book will ask you to begin by sitting comfortably on a flat surface—typically the floor—in a cross-legged position and with a straight spine. This is called Easy Pose. Try sitting on a blanket, a yoga mat, or a sheepskin for comfort. Adding a cushion directly under your "sit bones" can help you keep a straight spine and keep your hips higher than your knees. If you would rather sit in a chair, feel free to do so. Keep both feet flat on the ground with your weight distributed equally between them.

Where do I put my hands?

In yoga, hand positions are called *mudras*. These various positions are said to activate different *meridians*—the channels in the body through which the life energy called *chi* is thought to flow. Thus the positions are said to give distinct signals to your body, activating different glandular and nervous system activities. A common mudra, which is often seen in pictures of people meditating, is called *gyan mudra*. This mudra is done by touching the tip of the thumb to the tip of the index finger while holding the other fingers straight. Often, this mudra is used when you are sitting in Easy Pose, in which case, your elbows are straight and your wrists rest comfortably on your knees with the palms facing upward (see photo on page 37).

When I meditate, where do I focus my eyes?

Follow the directions of the particular meditation. If nothing is specified, close your eyes and focus at the point between your eyebrows.

What if my mind wanders?

People often say, "My mind is racing; I can't meditate," or "I forgot to focus." When you are meditating, your mind will ramble from thought to thought, from something that's worrying you to today's workload to your grocery list, and so on. Wonderful! This means you are meditating perfectly. This happens to advanced meditators too. Try simply to note the wandering and bring your mind gently back to the exercise. Don't push away thoughts; just let them dissipate or float away. Gently bring your mind back to the breath and the focus of the exercise. It's difficult but very calming to focus on the breath for greater periods of time.

Meditation, in a small way, gives you the chance to be a hero in your own story. The process of meditation causes many thoughts and emotions to fly at us constantly. The goal is to learn to hold on to what matters to you and stay steady. In fact, this is how you will know you are a good meditator: when all your thoughts come into your head, you gently thank them and choose instead to hold your attention steady. When you are meditating well, you continually and gently remind yourself to focus on the meditation and the present moment.

I feel a little strange after I meditate. Is that okay?

People sometimes feel light-headed after meditating, or parts of the body can feel numb or tingly. These are all normal feelings. After practicing, sit still for a bit. The light-headedness or tingly feelings are just your body and mind adjusting to the new techniques. Relax into them; they will pass in a few moments.

If you have questions that aren't answered here, try to accept that you don't know all the answers right now. If you gently contemplate your questions over time, you may find that you discover your own answers or that the question loses its urgency.

The Posture Is the Practice

In yoga, the posture is the practice—our minds and biochemistry work together with our posture to produce a state of well-being. Practicing yoga postures enables a deeper meditation because it creates a state of alert relaxation and directed attention. This can bring us into the present moment, facilitate a shift in mood, and lower anxiety. Yoga and meditation have another benefit as well: they create *radiance*, or *presence*.

Throughout the book, you will find that we use the terms "presence" and "radiance" interchangeably. That is because in Kundalini Yoga both terms are used to refer to this illusive quality.

Have you ever noticed at a meeting that when some people talk, everyone listens? Another person might say the exact same thing, and no one acknowledges it. Why is that? It has to do with the strength of their presence.

Anxiety interferes with presence because it takes you out of the current moment. Anxiety changes your posture—it makes you tense, awkward, or even slumped over, as your shoulders tighten. People with straighter postures are seen as more appealing than those who slouch (Mehrabian and Blum 1997). Slouching conveys a shut-down, uninviting body language to observers and makes the sloucher feel shut down as well.

Yoga and good posture require practice. If you practice straightening your posture throughout the day, the repetition will become part of your natural rhythm, and the effects will build steadily over time.

Developing this new practice will require some of that courage we talked about earlier and will take a bit of commitment on your part. Make a promise to yourself to try this new endeavor and invest in this process of change. As you develop your physical practice and it becomes integrated into your life, you'll find that your thoughts begin to change as well. You'll be better able to stay in the moment, allow negative thoughts to pop up and pass, and comfort yourself. Ultimately, this process will result in a reduction of anxiety, which will be replaced by a sense of authenticity that you can trust. This quality, which we call radiance, is the focus of Week 6, the final week of the Y-CBT program.

For now, let's start with yoga warm-ups, which will be part of your daily practice this week. As you embark on your new yoga practice, please remember to be mindful of any injuries or physical discomfort that you may experience, and adapt the movements accordingly.

Yoga Warm-Ups

These simple yoga warm-ups will help you become more flexible, both physically and mentally. Your spine will become suppler and your mind calmer. Some people report that their minds also seem to be more open to new possibilities after completing these exercises. Try each pose for the minimum specified time at first, then work your way to longer durations.

Throughout the yoga in this book you may notice that detailed instructions, such as how to hold your hands, are not always offered. This is because in the Kundalini Yoga tradition students are often encouraged to find their own way. Please remember that if no instructions are given about your eyes, you may close them.

KY YOGA:
Warm-Ups for a Flexible Spine
(M. K. Khalsa et al. 2014)

Sit in Easy Pose or in a chair, with your chest out and your shoulders back. Close your eyes.

1. (A) Put the palms of your hands on your knees.

    Deeply inhale as you flex your lower spine forward while lifting your chest.

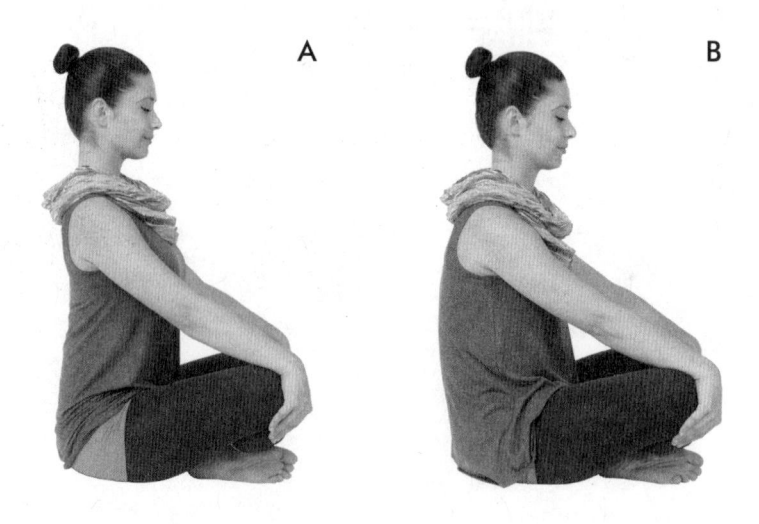

(B) Exhale as you flex your spine backward.

Keep your head level.

Repeat and continue.

Begin with 1 minute, and you can build to 3 minutes.

Relax the posture.

2. (C) Bring your hands to your shoulders with your fingers in front and thumbs in back.

   (D) Inhale as you twist left. Breathe in long and deep.

   (E) Exhale as you twist right.

   Repeat and continue for 1 minute, and you can build to 3 minutes.

   Relax the posture.

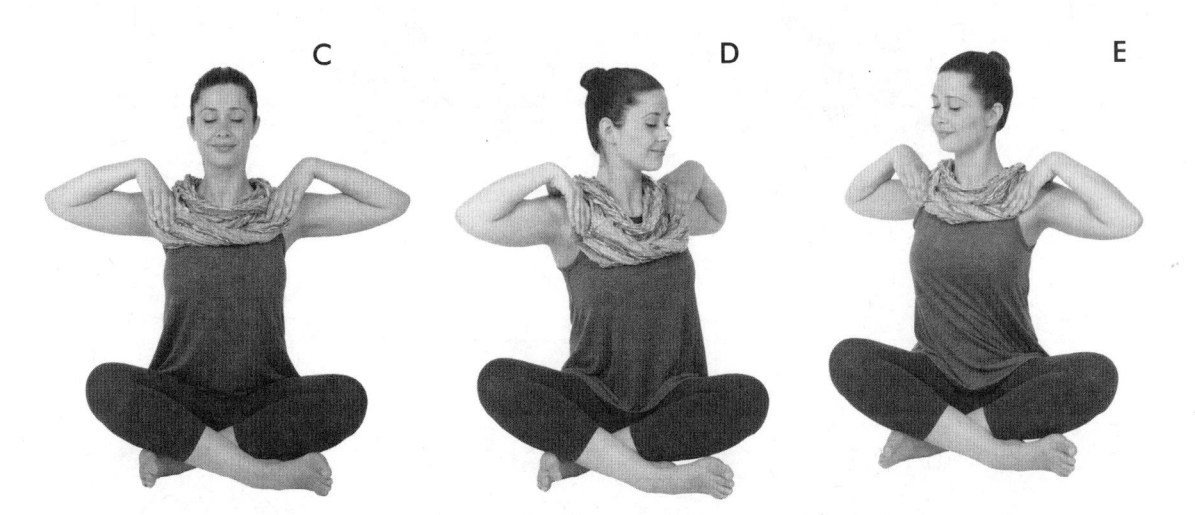

3. (F) Grasp your knees firmly, with your elbows straight.

   Inhale as you flex your upper spine forward.

   Exhale as you flex your upper spine backward.

   Repeat and continue.

   Begin with 1 minute, and you can build to 3 minutes.

   Relax the posture.

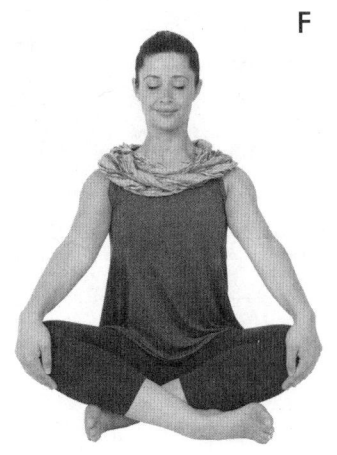

4. (G) Inhale as you shrug your shoulders up.

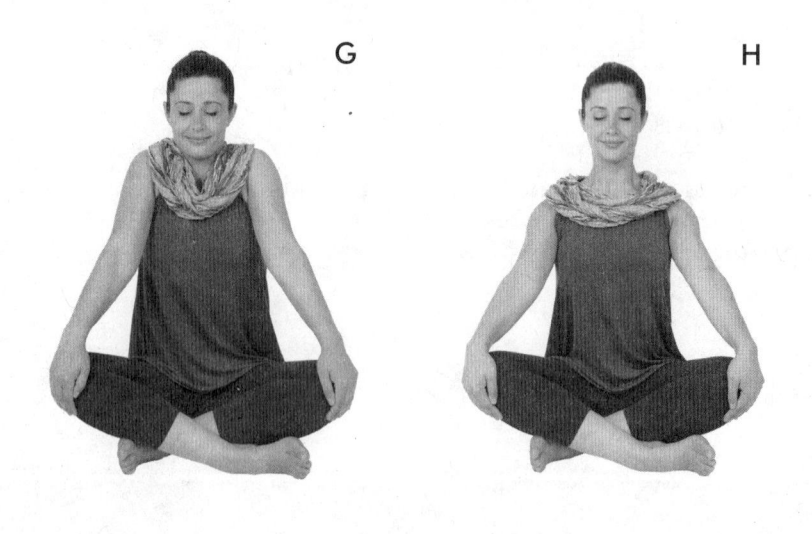

(H) Exhale as you shrug your shoulders down, still holding your knees.

Repeat and continue, moving at a relaxed pace.

Begin with 1 minute, and you can build to 2 minutes.

To end: Inhale and hold 15 seconds, with the shoulders held in a high shrug upward.

Relax the shoulders.

Inhale and suspend the breath briefly. Exhale and relax the breath, relax the posture.

As noted earlier, yoga sets are always followed by relaxation or meditation. After you do these warm-ups, we recommend you try the following Meditation on the Breath. This meditation will help you become aware of the physical and mental sensations created by the yoga warm-ups and will help you relax.

MEDITATION:
On the breath

Sit quietly and comfortably in Easy Pose.

Straighten your posture, with your shoulders over your hips, and your chest somewhat lifted.

Close your eyes and focus on the point between your eyebrows.

Place your hands in gyan mudra, resting on your knees with the palms facing upward.

Inhale and exhale through your nose. Allow your breath to relax and deepen.

Listen to the sound of your breath and the other sounds around you.

Notice the movement in your body as your breath lifts your chest.

Continue for 1 minute, and build to 3 minutes.

Inhale and suspend the breath briefly. Exhale and relax the breath, relax the posture.

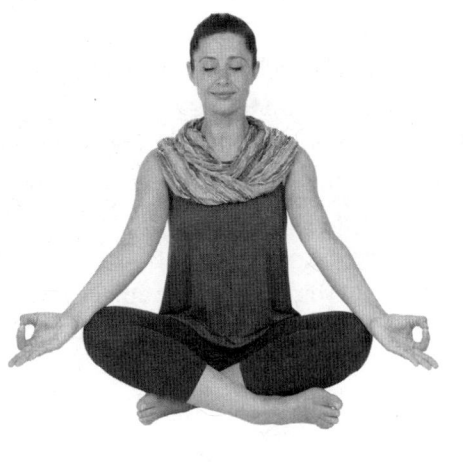

If you are ever in doubt about where to start your daily practice, the Warm-Ups for a Flexible Spine followed by the Meditation on the Breath are great choices. In fact, if you only have five minutes for your daily practice, just do these two things.

Attention in Action

Over time, a daily practice—even if it's just for a few minutes—will help you focus your attention and observe your thoughts and sensations. This process, called *attention in action*, can help you manage your anxiety by teaching you to stay in the present moment instead of being distracted by worries about the past or fears about the future. Attention in action is not just a part of your daily practice; it's a state of mind to cultivate throughout the day.

At any given moment, your mind might be caught up in one or more conversations with you. This can feel quite chaotic. When you are anxious, you may hear one part of your mind urging you to calm down so you can think more clearly. At the same time, another part of your mind may be experiencing a scary memory or a sensation of fear. Your body replicates your mood: your biochemistry alters, your muscles tighten, and your face reflects your anxious thoughts. This state of being is akin to driving a car while pressing on the gas pedal and the brakes at the same time. Obviously, there are better ways to drive a car—and to regulate a human mind and body.

Instead of passively giving in to a welter of conflicting thoughts, you can choose instead to actively focus your attention and *observe* your thoughts and sensations. If you do this compassionately, you will begin to see how and where your thoughts connect and relate to one another. In turn, this process will help you reduce your anxiety.

Attention in action draws upon three aspects of emotion and cognition: self-compassion, intention, and self-control.

Self-Compassion

Developing the practice of observing yourself with charity and benevolence is a form of *self-compassion*—a way of being kind to yourself. Expressing self-compassion can give you great resilience when you are challenged by your weaknesses or when you are confronted with your own personal difficulties.

Several studies have demonstrated the importance of self-compassion. Fillip Raes (2010) found that practicing self-compassion appeared to have a "cushioning effect" on depression and anxiety by reducing repetitive thinking, and Breines and Chen (2012) found that self-compassion increased motivation to improve personal weaknesses. Krieger and colleagues (2013) found that higher levels of self-compassion were related to lower levels of rumination and that, when compared with nondepressed people, depressed people showed lower levels of self-compassion.

Recent research has suggested that the practice of self-compassion may be an important component of success (Breines and Chen 2012), mindfulness (Van Dam et al. 2011), and happiness (Hollis-Walker and Colosimo 2011). Yoga and meditation can activate your ability for self-compassion.

EXERCISE:
Self-Compassion

This exercise will help you become more compassionate with yourself. Learning to extend the same kindness toward yourself as you do toward others will take practice. This exercise is your first step.

1. Sit quietly and comfortably in Easy Pose. Close your eyes.

2. Take a few deep breaths to center yourself.

3. Focus at the point between your eyebrows.

4. Consider a mistake that you have made recently, or some recent event that you have criticized yourself for.

5. Take a moment, and then open your eyes.

6. Write down the self-critical remark you said to yourself:

   _____

   _____

7. Choose a self-comforting or kind phrase of forgiveness that relates to the situation you have written about above. An example might be "I tried my best" or "I meant no harm." Write your comforting phrase here:

   _____

   _____

8. Return to taking long deep breaths and relaxing more deeply. Quietly repeat to yourself the comforting, self-compassionate phrase you have chosen. Notice how your body feels as you do this. Remember that you can choose to comfort yourself during hard times rather than repeat critical thoughts to yourself over and over.

9. Write how it felt to comfort rather than criticize yourself:

   _____

   _____

   _____

Shifting the way that you speak to yourself, and offering self-compassion rather then criticism, takes practice. If you are used to addressing yourself with harsh words, changing this process may seem strange at first. Learning to be self-supportive will teach you to notice your strengths and ultimately improve your self-confidence.

Intention

Pay attention to your intentions. *Intention* is what you want to achieve, like a purpose or a goal that matters to you. Anxiety often accompanies what we call an *innocent intention*, which is a simple wish common to all people, though we may not be consciously aware of it. For example, many of us experience intentions such as:

I want to fit in.

I want to be liked.

I want to succeed.

Anxiety is often linked to these intentions, because we are not sure if what we want is acceptable or achievable.

Though there is nothing inherently good or bad about any innocent intention, individuals who are anxious or depressed respond differently to them than people who are more confident and relaxed. The non-anxious person may respond to his or her intention with self-talk that is encouraging, kind, and supportive, while the person given to anxiety or depression may respond with hopelessness, criticism, and even condemnation.

If you can listen for, notice, and acknowledge your own innocent intentions, your anxiety will diminish. This happens because you are no longer fighting with your own truth.

In fact, anxiety can serve as a signal for you to pay attention to the quiet thoughts and feelings you might not be listening to. In this way, anxiety is like an olden-days farmhouse dinner bell: Once the cook finished cooking dinner, she rang the dinner bell on the porch to call the family. If everyone was nearby and responded right away, the cook only had to hit the bell briefly and not too loudly. But if folks didn't respond quickly, the cook would hit the bell harder and longer.

Just as a dinner bell signaled people to come home from the fields, anxiety may serve as a signal to pay attention to something you are trying to tell yourself. If you can listen to what is *beneath* the anxiety—the innocent intention—the anxiety will diminish. Acknowledging the truth of what you feel is liberating. The truth *does set you free,* because when you don't give all of your attention to fear you're able to pursue your intended goals. The next meditation will help you access your innocent intentions and come to accept and understand the feelings that are hidden by your fear and anxiety.

MEDITATION:
Attend to Your Intentions

1. Sit quietly and comfortably in Easy Pose. Close your eyes.

2. Take a few deep breaths to center yourself.

3. Focus at the point between your eyebrows. Observe your thoughts.

4. Take a moment, then open your eyes.

5. Write your thoughts here:

_____

_____

_____

_____

6. Continue taking long deep breaths and relaxing more deeply. As thoughts come up, try to hear the heart of the matter or the goal behind your thought. You can "befriend" the thought, accepting it with kindness and gratitude.

7. Write down what you discover. Are you any clearer on your intention? Can you respond to it with acceptance?

_____

_____

_____

_____

Knowing how to manage the fear and anxiety that keep your intentions hidden is a valuable skill. When you master it, your intentions will become much clearer to you. And once you understand them, the questions to ask yourself become: "Is this matter under my control? Or am I looking for something from someone else?"

Self-Control

Being in control of yourself requires placing your attention on what you can actually control—that is, your *own* self-talk, actions, and communications. Often, when people are feeling discomfort or unhappiness, they focus instead on the behavior or actions of others. Perhaps you spend a lot of mental energy reviewing what has happened during past conversations or imagining how things might go in the future: "Why did I say that to her? That was foolish, I made myself look stupid" followed by "Tomorrow she will call me out in front of everyone, and I will be the joke of the basketball team!" Do you ever have this type of dialogue in your mind?

Ultimately, we all have to admit that discussions in our heads, even if "directed" toward another person, are only conversations we are having with *ourselves*. These imagined discussions are usually not accurate or valid, and will not bring about change. In fact, this internal dialogue will only make you more anxious, simply because there is no input from the other person. The conversation consists only of your thoughts, typically coming from a negative perspective, *imagining* what the other person would say or do.

You can learn to shift your attention away from others and toward yourself. The following meditation is designed to help you do that. In turn, you will develop an authenticity that generates personal radiance.

EXERCISE:
Practicing Self-Control

Keep your attention on yourself in this exercise. Focus on and practice your ability to stay relaxed and calm. In the end, the best way to achieve your goals is by remaining calm and thinking clearly.

1. Sit quietly and comfortably in Easy Pose. Close your eyes.

2. Take a few deep breaths to center yourself.

3. Begin to still your body and relax into the posture.

4. Continue breathing deeply.

5. Focus on the point between your eyebrows.

6. Ask yourself, "Who am I trying to control? Is it me? Or am I trying to change the past or convince someone of something? What am I talking to myself about?" Write down your answer:

   _____

   _____

   _____

7. Ask yourself, "Am I physically calm?" Scan your body, particularly the places that are most affected by stress (head, chest, shoulders, back, and so forth). Ask, "How am I breathing? How can I shift my body's response to one of calm?" Write down your answer:

   _____

   _____

   _____

Remember, the best way to achieve your intentions is to become calm and relaxed. Did you discover that the more you could calm your body and release physical tension, the less anxious you felt? With a calmer physical body, can you more clearly see your intention?

We can't control other people (much as we might try). We can only control ourselves. By working with our attention, we can shift our focus to what we *can* change: our actions and our physical and emotional reactions to stress.

Working with Attention in Action

A tense mind and a tense body go together; relaxing one can relax the other. To alleviate anxiety, practice the following yoga set and broaden your focus to include more than one sense. Use deep breaths to allow or tolerate the presence of emotion. One of the poses asks for you to place your hands at your *heart center*. This is located at the center of your chest. The heart center represents compassion, kindness, and love.

It is said that the arm movements activate the meridians in the arms and hands, helping release old thought and feeling patterns that trigger fear and anxiety.

As noted earlier, in Kundalini Yoga and in Y-CBT a yoga set is always followed by a meditation or period of relaxation in order to reinforce and strengthen the benefits of the yoga. Be sure to read the yoga steps and the meditation all the way through before you begin. Familiarizing yourself with the steps and accompanying photographs will make the exercise go more smoothly.

This exercise has movement that is only on one side of the body. People often ask us why this is the case. The answer is that the human body is not symmetrical! The stomach, the liver, and the heart, for example, are only on one side, and so some exercises are specifically designed to target those unique areas.

Also, in the following exercise you'll notice that we ask you to move your arm forcefully. What do we mean by that? In KY the student finds his or her own rhythm and pace. While we are concerned with posture, KY is also concerned with the effort and consciousness that you put into the exercise. So please, in this and all exercises, set a pace that works for you.

KY YOGA:
Relief from Stress

(Bhajan and Khalsa 2000, 39)

Sit in Easy Pose. Close your eyes and focus on the center of your chin.

1. (A) Bend your right elbow so that your forearm is in front of your body with the palm facing down.

    Without bending your wrist, bend your arm at the elbow, moving your right hand up and down quickly from the tip of your nose to your navel.

    Move fast and forcefully. Put your entire self into the movement.

    Continue for 30 seconds. You can build to 1 minute.

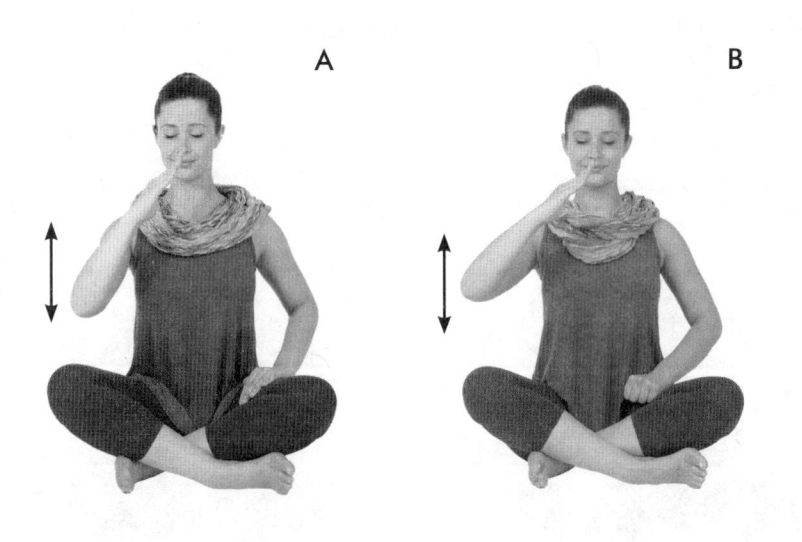

(B) Next, continue moving your right hand up and down, and make a tight fist with your left hand.

Continue the movement for 1 more minute. You can build to 2 minutes.

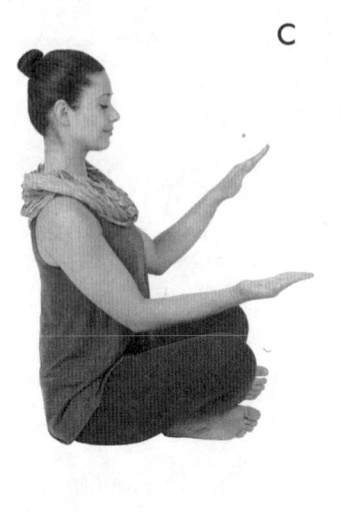

C

2. (C) Bring your arms down to your sides.

    Bend your elbows so that your forearms are parallel to the ground.

    The left palm faces down and right palm faces up.

    Move each forearm up and down alternately, moving powerfully.

    Continue the movement for 1.5 minutes. You can build to 3 minutes.

    The pace is 1 to 3 movements per second.

3. (D) Place your left hand flat against your chest on your heart center.

    Place your right hand on top of your left hand.

    Gently bend your neck to the left, bringing your left ear toward your left shoulder.

    Next, come back to a straight neck.

D

E

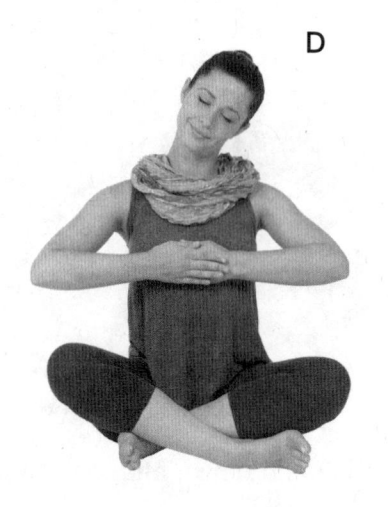 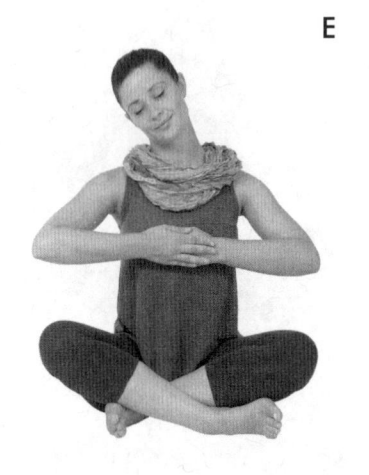

(E) Next, bend your neck to the right, bringing your right ear toward your right shoulder.

Next, come back to a straight neck.

Smoothly move your neck back and forth from the left position to the right position.

Repeat and continue for 1 minute, and you can build to 2 minutes.

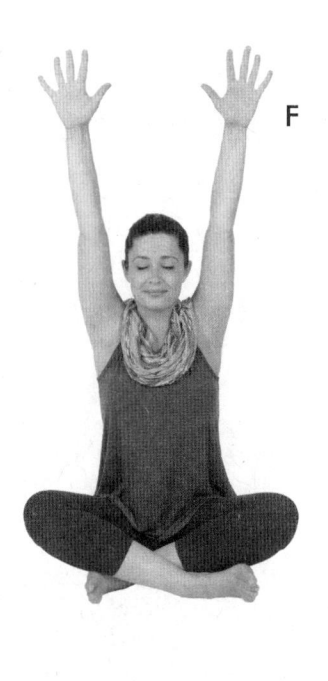

(F) Stretch your arms straight up over your head with the fingers open as wide as you can. Squeeze all of the muscles in your body as you stretch up.

Hold for 30 seconds. You can build to 1 minute.

Inhale and suspend the breath briefly. Exhale and relax the breath, relax the posture.

To remember: Stress is a natural part of life, and this set is said to help the glandular system adjust to stress.

How do you feel? This yoga set is designed to help relieve tension in your mind and body. You can do it anytime you are feeling particularly stressed. You can also add it to your daily practice.

The meditation described next will help calm your mind and relax your body. Use this meditation to stay focused on the present and create a calm center from which you can begin to choose your reactions to the world around you. The counting focuses your mind on your breath. This focus will help your mind remain engaged but relaxed. The counting is slow, and the breathing pattern will take all of your concentration. After doing this meditation, even for a just a few minutes, many people experience an increased sense of peace and feel as though their minds have been cleared of negative emotions from the past.

KY MEDITATION:
Stress Relief and Clearing Emotions of the Past

(Bhajan 1991)

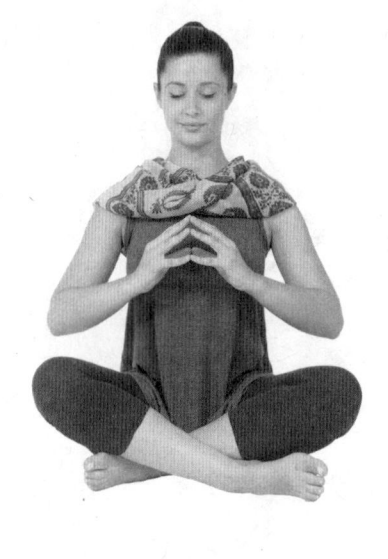

Sit in Easy Pose. Look at the tip of your nose.

Bring your hands together and lightly press the fingertips of one hand to your other hand, creating a space between the palms.

The fingers point upward, creating a tent.

Hold your hands in this position at the center of your chest.

Silently count to 5 as you:

  Inhale for 5 seconds.

  Hold your breath for 5 seconds.

  Exhale for 5 seconds.

Repeat and continue for 1 minute, and you can build to 11 minutes.

Inhale and suspend the breath briefly. Exhale and relax the breath, relax the posture.

To remember: This meditation is especially helpful for dealing with stressful relationships and with past family issues. If your mind wanders, gently bring it back to the counting.

For most people, establishing a daily practice is not easy, as it requires significant life and attitude changes. However, a daily practice leads to positive and usually profound life changes for just about everyone who commits to it with dedication.

Week 1 Daily Y-CBT Practice

Guiding Principle

Everyone is capable of great courage and has a remarkable ability to change. Each person can create a calm place from which they can constructively face their thoughts, emotions, and relationships.

Yoga and Meditation

1. Yoga Warm-Ups for a Flexible Spine

2. Stress Relief and Clearing Emotions of the Past

3. One other meditation to work with self-compassion, attending to your intentions, or gaining self-control

Practice each pose and meditation for a minimum of 1 minute each.

Daily Living Practice

This week you will learn about creating a daily yoga and meditation practice to develop your ability to manage anxiety. Notice how you feel about the idea of having a daily yoga and meditation practice.

Ask yourself, "What's required to have a daily practice? What must shift in my life—mentally and logistically?" Remind yourself that you have the courage and ability to change.

During the week, apply these techniques and principles as you go through your day:

*   Observe your thoughts and sensations, along with where you focus your attention.

*   Practice attention in action—taking hold of your attention to reduce anxiety.

*   Practice self-compassion.

*   Accept and listen to your intentions. Refer back to the Attend to Your Intentions meditation when you need a refresher.

*   Remember that we can't control other people. We can only control ourselves. Do the Practicing Self-Control exercise if you notice your attention wavering from yourself to others.

Daily Practice Log

It's very helpful to keep track of the techniques you are using and your progress. Use this log to do that. Using a scale of 1 to 10, rate your anxiety *before* you try the technique. Practice the technique, and then rate your anxiety *after* you finish.

	Sunday		Monday		Tuesday		Wednesday		Thursday		Friday		Saturday	
Time of Day														
	B	A	B	A	B	A	B	A	B	A	B	A	B	A
Yoga/Meditation I Used														
Y-CBT Techniques I Used														

B = Before, A = After

1	2	3	4	5	6	7	8	9	10
Low Anxiety				Moderate Anxiety				High Anxiety	

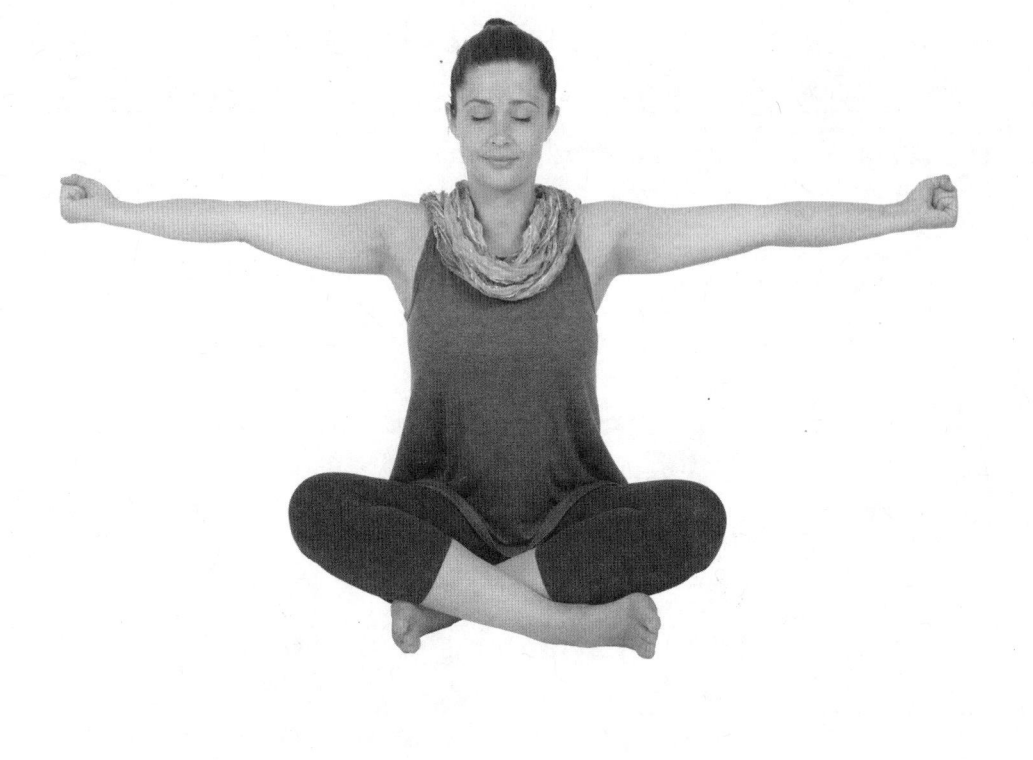

WEEK 2

Working with Anxiety and Panic

A s mentioned, anxiety can be caused by a current situation or triggered by a thought or stimulus, such as a certain smell or sound, that reminds you of something unpleasant from your past. Whatever the trigger, the fear response created by anxiety has a dramatic effect on your thoughts and your physical state.

A variety of biochemical changes in your body, fueled by your memories and imagination, combine to produce many symptoms of anxiety, which have both physical and cognitive (mental) components.

Cognitive (Thoughts) Symptoms of Anxiety

Unstoppable, ruminative negative thoughts

Worry (unfounded or exaggerated fears)

Dread of a place or thing

Frightening images

A generalized fear of the past or the future

Panicky beliefs that everything is going wrong

Physical Symptoms of Anxiety

Restlessness

Tingling in the extremities

Muscle tension

Light-headedness

Sleeplessness

Rapid heart rate

Sweating

In this chapter, we will explore Y-CBT guiding principle number two: **The mind and body are fluidly connected.**

This principle is based on the idea that the state of the mind is dependent on the state of the body, and vice versa. As one shifts, the other will follow in kind. In the coming pages, we will teach you about this connection and how to develop a *positive* relationship between your mind and body. As you integrate this guiding principle into *your* belief system and work with the associated techniques, you will be able to better identify both your physical and thought reactions to anxiety and panic, and learn how to resolve them more effectively.

Anxiety Is a Mind-Body Experience

As we have discussed, anxiety has two distinct sets of symptoms: some occur within your mind (cognitively) as thoughts, and some happen in your body as physical reactions. Often the combined impact is so intertwined that it isn't easy to notice your multifaceted reaction.

There are two key factors in fully managing anxiety:

- To become aware of how anxiety impacts both your mind and your body

- To recognize that the sensations that happen in one will automatically put the other into action: *The mind and body are fluidly connected.*

Learning to become *aware* of the constant interplay between your thoughts and your physical responses is an important step in managing the symptoms of your unique experience.

Fear activates the body's natural alarm system. When there is a real danger—such as a fire, a burglar, or a wild animal—the body's various systems automatically spring into action. Your nervous system, your brain, and your biochemistry quickly assess the situation, and, in many instances, you will physically move away from the source of fear. Once the actual danger has passed, your body will return to its normal state with time.

When we experience *emotional* fear or anxiety, our body reacts the same way it does when there is an actual threat, but frequently we are unable to accurately assess and resolve the situation and then calm our body and mind. Your mind reacts to the complexities of your fear, and your body reacts to your stressful thoughts. This might mean that your shoulders tense up or your stomach ties up in knots. At first, you might not notice the physical response, because you are engulfed by what is going on in your mind. Left unchecked, the body becomes increasingly agitated, leading to a higher baseline state of stress, or what you get used to feeling on a day-to-day basis.

Sometimes symptoms of anxiety first arise in your body, and then your mind reacts. You might bolt awake in the middle of the night with a racing heart, or you might begin to shake the minute you walk into a meeting. Very often, when the body initiates the sequence, the mind begins to match the physical symptoms with a litany of negative thoughts or images, and you might begin to worry about what challenging or stressful things are about to happen.

As your mind sorts through the complexities of the fears, your body is reacting to the effects of your thoughts. Perhaps you recognize this cycle: when your body is experiencing the physical symptoms of anxiety, your mind begins to ruminate or even obsess. Quieting *both* aspects of anxiety is crucial to getting a complete resolution. That's where Y-CBT comes in. Y-CBT seeks to break this ping-pong cycle by simultaneously addressing the physical *and* cognitive symptoms of anxiety.

We all have our own biochemical predisposition and vulnerability to a particular level of anxiety—that initial spontaneous response we have to anything that scares us. In other words, individuals differ in how intensely they respond to stress, how fast their hearts race, and how much anxiety they feel in a stressful situation. Yoga and meditation can be particularly helpful in reducing the intense, initial stage of anxiety, because yoga and meditation have been shown to affect the hormonal and nervous systems that allow you to respond with lowered reactivity to such situations (Gard et al. 2014).

Anxiety in the Mind

In our minds, anxiety takes the form of a rapid succession of fear-based thoughts. Worry and rumination—that repetitive loop of negative thinking—is something everyone has experienced. These thoughts might be triggered by a fact or an actual event. When driven by anxiety, the thought process can magnify a difficult situation, turning it into an unreasonable version of the original concern.

Perhaps you've found yourself saying, "I've gone over the problem a million times, and it just gets worse in my mind," or "I'm exhausted because my mind never stops," or "I'm thinking about everything all the time."

This type of thinking is the anxious mind's attempt to manage the source of the fear. Whether this fear is internal (a thought about the past or the future) or external (a stressful event), once we start to experience anxiety, our minds begin a process of attempting to manage the experience by moving into overdrive and perpetually thinking about and rehashing the problem again and again.

This anxious response to fear is ineffective; in fact, it often brings on more distress. Anxiety brings with it emotions and irrational fears about people, places, and things, and, for the time being, shuts out the possibility of constructive problem solving. The mind can also race, or even create panic, about a past event or anticipated problems in the future.

In the mind, anxiety can manifest as any of the following:

Generalized fear	Feelings of terror	Apprehension
Overthinking	Frightening images	Irrational fears
Racing thoughts	Insecurity	Confusion
Unstoppable thoughts	Dwelling on the past	Fear of the future
Worry or dread	Flashbacks	
Rumination	Agitated thoughts	

While some anxious people feel chronically apprehensive, or may begin each day with a sense of dread without a clear idea of what is driving the feelings, most anxious feelings are accompanied by worry. Worry involves illogical chains of thoughts and language that keep the mind very busy. This process is different than logical, fact-based problem solving.

Worry often paints a fear-driven picture of the future. It occupies our minds in an often nonproductive process of remaining engaged with the source of fear. Have you ever mulled over a feared event and thought of all the possible negative outcomes, down to the very last detail? This type of ruminative worry is common. This process fools you into believing that you're doing something about a problem when, in reality, you're doing nothing but filling your mind with a heightened level of negative thoughts. Because your mind is busy, you might *feel* that you're working toward a solution, but actually you are probably just going around in circles and getting nowhere!

Worry is such a central component of the anxious mind that we will examine this cognitive feature more fully in the next chapter.

Anxiety in the Body

One of the most disturbing aspects of anxiety is how many of the body's critical systems are affected. Anxiety impacts the cardiovascular, nervous, and respiratory systems. These disruptions create *extrapyramidal symptoms*, or those related to motor activity, such as shaking, muscle weakness, or tingling.

When we are anxious, our heart rate and blood pressure increase (Dimitriev, Saperova, and Dimitriev 2016), and this can lead to an experience of a racing, pounding heart. These blood-flow changes can cause headaches and tingling in the hands or the feeling of wobbly legs.

The nervous system puts the body on high alert when we are anxious, shutting down some systems and activating others. The sympathetic nervous system, for example, releases adrenaline to prepare the body for action (Bourne 2015), causing us to feel nervous, shaky, or jittery. Many changes take place in the brain (Dimitriev, Saperova, and Dimitriev 2016), and the default mode network may be activated, bringing on rumination, anxiety, and depression, which we'll discuss in greater detail later in this chapter.

In normal breathing, the nervous system determines the depth and frequency of the breath to balance the supply of carbon dioxide and oxygen in the blood. We breathe in oxygen for our cells to use in producing energy. The breathing process creates the natural by-product carbon dioxide, which is expelled when we exhale. When we are anxious, our respiratory rate changes (Dimitriev, Saperova, and Dimitriev 2016). Anxiety can result in hyperventilation, which causes feelings of light-headedness and faintness (Greenberger and Padesky 1995).

Anxiety and the Breath

When people experience fear or extreme anxiety, their breathing patterns change. Sometimes people momentarily hold their breath, or, at other times, their rate of breathing might increase. These reactions can create abnormal levels of carbon dioxide in the blood. This irregularity in the levels of carbon dioxide triggers symptoms of light-headedness, palpitations, sweating, and numbness which confuse the body, making it feel as though it may be suffocating,. The body then naturally goes on high alert, causing a survival response physically, emotionally, and cognitively. Altogether, these actions create a negative sequence: the breath is held, the mind races, and the heart races.

Let's look at how problematic this sequence is for Laura, who experiences the sudden, seemingly unexplainable onset of social anxiety. One day Laura was enjoying a pleasant lunch with her former college roommate. Every year for their birthdays, which are only days apart, they meet at a beautiful restaurant in Boston. On this afternoon, during dessert, Laura heard a sigh and saw what she thought was a dismissive gesture from her companion that made her feel insecure. Laura wondered: "Did I say something wrong? Why is she looking at me like that?" She began to imagine that her friend wanted to leave because she had become tired of her company. Laura went into an emotional tailspin and found herself flooded with more anxious thoughts, feelings, and physical reactions. "She doesn't like me after all. She only came today because she had to…" As her thoughts progressed, Laura's hands began to shake, she felt dizzy, and her heart began to pound. She reached for her water glass and spilled it on the table. Humiliated, Laura ran from the room.

What happened to Laura? She began having negative anxious thoughts triggered by an unfounded fear. As her thoughts escalated, her body began to react, too, experiencing some of these common anxious breath patterns:

- Sudden sucking in of the breath

- Holding the breath

- Taking quick, short, shallow breaths

- Exhaling through the mouth

These reactions caused abnormalities in Laura's respiratory system, including irregularities in her carbon dioxide levels. Laura's inefficient breathing patterns contributed to many of her physical symptoms associated with anxiety, such as shaking, heart pounding, and light-headedness.

If, in the moment, Laura had taken a deep breath instead of holding her breath, she might have been able to relax her body and then take a moment to quiet the illogical negative thoughts by noting that all was well and that her friend had simply sighed.

Research has begun to support the notion that different breathing patterns and anxiety go hand in hand (Roth 2005). But the good news is this: breathing more effectively is something we can learn to control, and doing so has been shown to affect anxiety (Paulus 2013). To begin our study of the breath, let's start with what it means to breathe a simple natural breath.

Natural Breathing

Simple Natural Breathing is unfamiliar to many anxious people, although this is the kind of breath we are born with. This breath engages the diaphragm muscle, a partition separating the chest organs from the abdomen that is central to the process of respiration.

To try this breath, sit comfortably, either cross-legged on the floor or in a chair with both feet on the ground; alternatively, you may choose to lie on your back. Close your eyes and place your hands on your stomach. Allow the breath to come in and go out through the nose. Feel your stomach rise as you inhale and fall as you exhale. This swelling and subsiding is caused by the rise and fall of the diaphragm. As you breathe in this way, the lungs will naturally follow the movement of the diaphragm.

In Y-CBT, we have a variation on simple Natural Breathing that we call the Walking Around Breath. We encourage people to practice this breath as often as possible as they go about their day—you could be in your car, walking the halls at work, or preparing a meal. Those who do it report that the technique lowers anxiety and creates calm.

To try Walking Around Breath, use your diaphragm as in simple Natural Breathing. Relax your breath. Inhale and exhale through the nose about five times per minute (six seconds per inhale, followed by a six-second exhale). Note that breathing through the nose tends to be more calming than mouth breathing. In fact, mouth breathing or gulping air can be a symptom of anxiety and may exacerbate other physiological symptoms. Practicing Walking Around Breath for even one minute will generate noticeable change—and practicing for several minutes will calm you even further.

Basic Yoga Breath

Long Deep Breathing is a basic yoga breath from the tradition of Kundalini Yoga, but it is common in many different yoga practices. It's a deep, diaphragmatic breath that will help relax your body, quiet your mind, and calm your emotions. It is an excellent resource in moments of stress.

When you are overwhelmed, anxious, or worried, the *sympathetic nervous system* is in control. As long as this excitatory system is in charge, it's virtually impossible to get relief. The way to counter that is to put the calming *parasympathetic nervous system* in control. With Long Deep Breathing, you can actually begin to make this switch on your own and calm yourself down when needed.

Spicuzza and colleagues (2000) found that the action of diaphragmatic breathing reduced the neurological activation of the sympathetic nervous system. In other words, taking a deep breath triggers your nervous system to lower the activity of this excitatory system, which is associated with a cascade of biochemicals related to anxiety. Just by taking a long deep breath, you can learn to prevent anxiety symptoms! You'll have an immediate feeling of relief, though it can take time for the rest of your body to fully quiet down, as the parasympathetic nervous system starts to takes over. So the more long deep breaths you can take, the better. You may still have to face difficult circumstances, but the breath will give you the opportunity to consider the issues you face from a calmer, more aware place.

Long Deep Breathing is "the foundation of your yoga practice," according to Hari Kaur Khalsa (2015), a renowned trainer of yoga teachers and coauthor of *A Woman's Book of Yoga* (2002).

Long Deep Breathing can be done as a meditation, or it can be done at any time, in any place. Even when there's stress all around you, this breath will help calm your mind and body. When you're anxious, slow breathing can help inhibit sympathetic nervous system activity while also increasing the activity of the parasympathetic nervous system, with its calming effects (Jerath et al., 2015). Practicing Long Deep Breathing when stressed is like taking a cool drink of water on a hot summer day.

KY MEDITATION:
Long Deep Breathing

(Bhajan 2003, 92)

Sit in Easy Pose with your hands in gyan mudra (see Week 1).

Bring your attention to how your breath feels as it goes in and out, and as it fills and empties your lungs.

Hear the sound and feel the movement of your body as you deeply breathe in and out. Feel the center of your stomach as it expands and relaxes with the breath.

Close your eyes and focus at the point between your eyebrows.

Inhale slowly through your nose. Expand your stomach, then your chest. Exhale and relax your stomach and lungs.

Repeat and continue the sequence.

Begin with 1 minute, and you can build to 11 minutes.

Inhale and suspend the breath briefly. Exhale and relax the breath, relax the posture.

To remember: This is a long, slow deep breath that will fill you with oxygen, relax you, and open your mind to seeing things in new ways. Relax your stomach, chest, and shoulders. When you finish this meditation, take a moment to notice how you are feeling. When you are ready, bring your awareness back to your surroundings, and open your eyes.

When you meditate, all kinds of stray thoughts will come up. That's good; it means that you are meditating well. Just observe the thoughts and gently go back to focusing on the breath. As Yogi

Bhajan said, "If we can practically control the breath in such a way that it is normal and simple and soft, man in behavior will be normal, simple and soft" (1970).

Long Deep Breathing helps unite body and mind. As you focus on your breathing, you will naturally notice your body's response. Observing the experience of your thoughts and your breath from a neutral place offers you the quiet, peaceful experience of that unity.

Throughout the coming days, notice your breath: How fast are you breathing? Are you breathing through your nose or your mouth? Do you breathe differently when you are anxious than when you are calm?

Remember that excess carbon dioxide confuses the body into thinking it's suffocating and triggers rapid, shallow breathing, which keeps the cycle going! Moreover, this may lead to additional physical symptoms of anxiety, and sometimes panic attacks will ensue. Learning to control and improve your breath will ultimately restore normal levels of carbon dioxide in your bloodstream, which will help decrease your symptoms of anxiety.

So when you find yourself in life's difficult moments, take a deep breath and gently tell yourself, "I'll take a deep breath, and I'll be okay!"

Panic

The most extreme example of how anxiety affects the body is the panic attack. A panic attack is a brief, discrete experience of extreme anxiety resulting in dramatic physical symptoms that can last three to ten minutes. Symptoms typically include a racing heart, tremulousness, nausea, shortness of breath, dizziness, numbness, and tingling of the extremities. Some people report that these symptoms appear to come out of the blue, and they can be so extreme that they can be mistaken for a heart attack or stroke (American Psychiatric Association 2013). A panic attack can leave people feeling as though their bodies are completely out of control. This overpowering physical event commonly leads to extreme and catastrophic thoughts in the mind.

The Effect of Panic on the Body

Panic is thought to be triggered by the physiological fear response that occurs during a real or perceived danger or threat. When a person experiences fear, the brain sends a message to the autonomic nervous system. This message engages the sympathetic nervous system, which triggers the fight-or-flight response, preparing the body to either battle or run from the threat. Normally, once the threat has passed, the parasympathetic nervous system is activated by the brain, and calm is restored within the body (Li and Stamatakis 2011; Bourne 2015).

Panic attacks seem to occur when this system of activation and restored calm is not working effectively (Barlow and Craske 2007). Current research has begun to show that yoga and meditation affect parasympathetic activity, in part by reducing emotional reactivity and the autonomic nervous system responses associated with heightened emotion. This seems to hold true immediately following a yoga practice, and it appears that, over time, sustained yoga practice has the capacity to shift the body's baseline reactivity, so that it takes more stress to throw us off balance (Gard et al. 2014).

Panic attacks may also stem from abnormal breathing patterns that lead to an imbalance of carbon dioxide in the bloodstream (Bourne 2015). People who experience panic attacks report feeling that they can't get enough air. To compensate, people try to overbreathe, resorting to a rapid, shallow breathing from the chest and often through the mouth. This can lead to frightening symptoms such as dizziness, rapid heartbeat, and tingling in the arms and legs.

Research also suggests that some people may produce higher levels of adrenaline or other chemicals in their bodies, owing to chronic stress or other circumstances. These chemical imbalances lead to a constant state of mild or moderate physical stress. Eventually, the chronic imbalance reaches a level that triggers the dramatic fear response that leads to a panic attack. To the person experiencing such an attack, it seems to have occurred for no clear reason, out of the blue (Barlow and Craske 2007).

The Effect of Panic on the Mind

If you have experienced a panic attack, no one has to tell you that the physical symptoms can be terrifying. Fear is the appropriate human response when your body is out of control for unknown reasons.

When a person experiences fear, the mind seeks a logical cause for these intense feelings. When no good explanation is at hand, thoughts of doom and devastation can follow: "I am going to die. I am going crazy. I am out of control." It becomes impossible to concentrate or think straight.

This cascade of catastrophic, reactive, and fear-driven beliefs escalates the body's response. As mentioned, abnormal breathing only compounds the physical symptoms, triggering more frightened thoughts and leading to a negative cycle between the mind and the body.

Panic Attack Facts

Information is powerful, and equipping yourself with the facts about panic attacks can help you deal with them:

- *A panic attack typically lasts only three to ten minutes.* People who struggle with panic disorder will often say that their panic attacks last for hours at a time or even for days at a time. The fact is, the acute phase of a panic attack, with its profound physical symptoms, lasts only three to ten minutes. That's because, when left to its natural progression, the autonomic nervous system quickly sends a message to the parasympathetic system, which restores calm in the body.

  If you struggle with panic attacks, you can prove this to yourself with this simple action: When the panic begins, find a quiet place to sit and focus on the second counter on your wristwatch or phone. Make this counter your focal point. This simple action will help regulate your breathing, distract you from the symptoms, and prove to you exactly how long it takes for the acute symptoms to subside. The acute panic event will pass quickly. And remember, a panic attack will not kill you, you aren't going crazy, and gradually your body will come back into control.

- *A panic attack is exacerbated by and may even be caused by abnormal carbon dioxide levels in the blood.* A growing body of research suggests that an important feature of panic is inadequate regulation of the respiratory function. The key to stopping the acute phase of a panic attack is to restore normal levels of carbon dioxide in the blood. In one study, researchers successfully taught participants how to take control of their breathing patterns and alter their exhaled carbon dioxide levels (Meuret et al. 2008).

- *Paying attention to your breath can avert a panic attack.* Paulus (2013) suggests that calm people may be more sensitive to changes in their breathing patterns and thus may adapt more quickly in stressful situations by correcting the pattern earlier and more easily than anxious people do. If you struggle with anxiety, you may be less attuned to these subtle changes in your breath, so your breathing patterns may more easily become extreme and erratic, resulting in the experience of panic.

In the following section, you will learn two breath techniques that will help you address the regulation of oxygen and carbon dioxide in your body. In our practice, we have found that a particular type of breath work (Antidote Breath, see below) is found to be most helpful during the acute phase of panic, and it's easy to learn.

Breath Techniques for Working with Acute Panic

One of the most frightening symptoms of a panic attack is the sensation of suffocation. This symptom is the direct result of irregular levels of carbon dioxide in the bloodstream caused by abnormal breathing, such as over-breathing or shallow breathing. As we have noted, we breathe in oxygenated air and breathe out the waste product that includes carbon dioxide gas.

One method that may help regulate the level of carbon dioxide in the blood is to inhale through the nose and exhale through the mouth through pursed lips. In medical settings, this technique is called *pursed-lip breathing*, and it involves a shorter inhale and a longer exhale (Cabral et al. 2015). The technique is used with people who have breathing problems such as chronic obstructive pulmonary disease (COPD), because it helps to reduce the carbon dioxide in the blood (Cabral et al. 2015). Our colleague John Boisseau suggests a form of pursed-lip breathing informally known as Smell the Roses, Blow Out the Candles. He suggests that this technique may be helpful for people who struggle with panic attacks just as it is for those who suffer from COPD.

We have taken the basics of this breath, added counting, and renamed it the Antidote Breath for you to use specifically for managing an acute panic attack. As the name suggests, this breath may help you regain control and reverse the symptoms of a panic attack. Simply having a plan—and knowing what to do when a panic attack strikes—may reduce a panic attack's magnitude and your feelings of being out of control.

If you follow the instructions for this technique while in the grip of an acute panic attack, you may be able to restore normal respiratory patterns. Within a few breaths, the sensation of suffocation may start to decrease, and within a few minutes it may be gone altogether. A good way to master this technique is to practice while you are *not* having a panic attack.

EXERCISE:
Antidote Breath

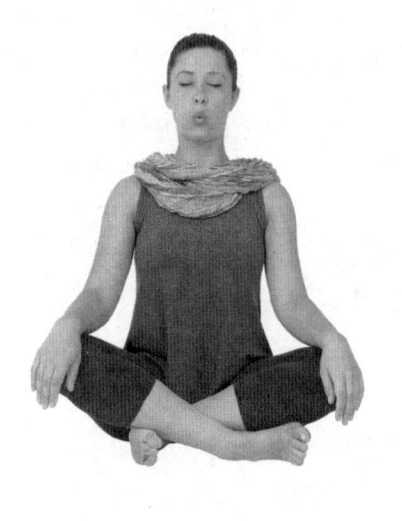

You can immediately address the symptoms of a panic attack by changing your breathing pattern. Practice this breath periodically when you are *not* having a panic attack so you feel comfortable doing it when you do feel the onset of panic.

Purse your lips into a pucker.

Inhale through your nose for a count of 3.

Then exhale through your mouth for a count of 6.

Continue for 3 or 4 breaths, or until the acute symptoms are reduced.

In our work, we have discovered interesting overlaps between the techniques of modern therapeutic practice and those of ancient traditions. The Antidote Breath, borrowed from Western medicine, closely resembles the following Silent Listening Within meditation, which comes from ancient yogic traditions. This meditation is very helpful for calming and quieting both the physical and emotional aspects of anxiety, because it too may help reestablish a healthy oxygen–carbon dioxide balance in your body.

A key element in many meditation practices is the focus on the breath. One study indicates that meditators are more accurate in interpreting respiratory signals or changes than are non-meditators (Daubenmier et al. 2013). Regular meditation practice can make you more attuned to changes in your normal breathing patterns. As you become more familiar with these patterns, you will be better able to notice and correct the shallow breathing that precedes the onset of a panic attack.

KY MEDITATION:
Silent Listening Within

(Bhajan 1995)

Sit calmly in Easy Pose with a straight spine.

Close your eyes if you wish.

Place your left hand flat against the chest with the right palm flat on top of the left. Both thumbs rest on the chest, pointing up and extending toward the chin.

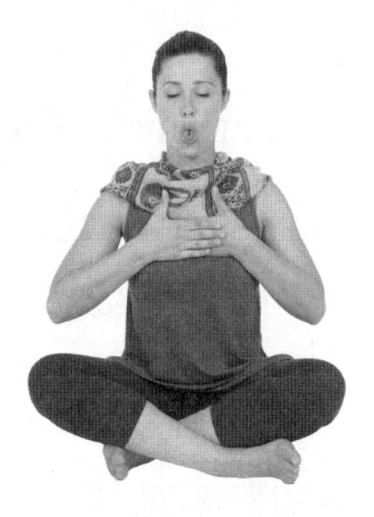

Open your mouth slightly with puckered lips.

Extend your tongue a little beyond the lips, and curl it into a "U" shape if you are able (*sitali pranayam*).

Inhale through your nose and exhale through your rolled tongue.

Repeat and continue this breathing pattern.

Begin with 1 to 3 minutes, and build up to 31 minutes.

Inhale and suspend the breath briefly. Exhale and relax the breath, relax the posture.

Think of the Antidote Breath and the Silent Listening Within meditation as tools in your anxiety management tool kit. Incorporate them into your daily practice or use them anytime you are experiencing symptoms of panic. You only need a quiet place and a few minutes to practice them. Most people find that the more often they practice these techniques, the more skilled they are in using them when needed, and the quicker the panic subsides.

Aftermath and Anticipatory Anxiety

People often report that their panic attacks go on for hours and sometimes even days. You now understand that an acute panic attack lasts only a very short time. However, the discomfort of the actual panic attack causes a prolonged fear after the acute phase is over and then extends to a belief that a panic attack can happen again at any time. Combined, these factors create thoughts and beliefs that can make it seem as though the panic attack is continuing all day long. By addressing the aftermath fear and the anticipation of the next panic attack as anxiety experiences *separate from* the acute panic attack, you will achieve greater control over your physical and emotional state.

Aftermath Anxiety

Aftermath anxiety is the response that follows the acute panic attack. Given the profound discomfort and terror that people feel during a panic attack, it is only natural that fear and trepidation would continue to dominate their thoughts after the acute symptoms have passed. Thoughts of dread and doom remain as people think about what they have just experienced:

I thought I was going to die.

My heart nearly exploded.

I think I burst a blood vessel in my head.

As these thoughts continue to roll, the traumatic experience of the acute event is reinforced and reexperienced, prolonging the physical effects. In other words, you can remain connected to the panic event in a state of fear *after* the acute event is over. Remember, this continued state of fear is triggering the physiological responses in the brain to respond and defend. Therefore, the state of the body remains agitated and the breath is shallow and insufficient, which is what makes it seem as if the panic attack is continuing beyond the acute event.

Anticipatory Anxiety

It is also common and reasonable to anticipate when the next panic attack will occur. It is a natural human response to prepare oneself for a frightening event. However, thinking about the next attack causes you to remain in a constant state of fear known as *anticipatory anxiety* and to live in a state of hypervigilance as an attempt to be alert for the next attack. This anticipatory pattern of thought drives a negative mind-body cycle. The insidiousness of the pattern is that repeating these fear-based thoughts can trigger the physiological response again, thus increasing the likelihood of *another* acute event:

I know that I will have a panic attack if I go to the grocery store.

I'll never get my work done because I will have a panic attack.

If I can't pay my bills, I will have a panic attack.

The next panic attack will surely kill me.

The fear of having a panic attack and the process of anticipating or preparing for the next one constitutes a perceived danger. As the thoughts predict the probability of the next event, the autonomic nervous system prepares the body to respond, resulting in more anxiety.

Addressing Aftermath and Anticipatory Anxiety

Recognizing the cycle of panic is key to managing and reducing the symptoms and frequency of the attacks. If you have struggled with panic attacks, your state of mind and the beliefs you have developed over time are what drive the problematic effects of aftermath and anticipatory anxiety. The fear-based belief system triggers the physiological response to defend and protect.

The symptoms of aftermath and anticipatory anxiety can be addressed with techniques that differ from those we offered you for managing an acute panic attack (see the following table). As we have learned, addressing acute panic requires normalizing the level of carbon dioxide in the body, as described earlier in the Antidote Breath and Silent Listening Within sections. Anticipatory and aftermath anxiety are best treated with a steady calming breath, such as Long Deep Breathing, which provides a balanced oxygen flow. In addition, it's important to address your thoughts, calming and quieting them with facts, which will help your body to stop reacting with a fear response. You can work with your thoughts by using the Powering Down to Transform Anxiety meditation or Set for Clear Thinking yoga, which is explained in the following section.

Learning to proactively address and change your panic cycle by targeting your fear responses as they occur and before they accelerate will lead to an overall reduction of the states of agitation and hypervigilant readiness.

Differences Between an Acute Panic Attack and Its Other Phases

	Acute Panic Attack	Aftermath Anxiety	Anticipatory Anxiety
Symptoms	breathlessness, racing heart, pounding head, dizziness, tremulousness, terror	shallow breathing, holding of the breath, fear, racing mind, rumination	shallow breathing, holding of the breath, fear, racing mind, predicting the future, self-defeating planning
Help: Work with your mind	"This will be over soon. I can watch my watch: just three minutes. I'm not dying; I just have to normalize my carbon dioxide levels by regulating my breathing."	"I'm okay. I can calm myself and focus on my breath. The panic attack happened but it is over now."	"I'll be okay. I know how to handle an attack. And I can breathe and focus on my breath. I can have greater control of how my body reacts to fear."
Help: Work with your breath and posture	Antidote Breath (inhale through the nose, exhale through the mouth) and Silent Listening Within	Long Deep Breathing (inhale through the nose, exhale through the nose) or One-Minute Breath (inhale, hold, exhale)	Long Deep Breathing (inhale through the nose, exhale through the nose) or One-Minute Breath (inhale, hold, exhale)

Thinking clearly is key to managing aftermath and anticipatory anxiety. The following yoga set is believed to impact the frontal lobe of the brain, which is the seat of many functions, including clear, calm thinking. This set can help improve the executive functioning of the brain, which will help to foster clearer thinking.

KY YOGA:
Set for Clear Thinking
(Bhajan 1983a, 52)

1. (A) Sit in Easy Pose.

    Place your hands on your knees.

    Begin vibrating the front of your face with a short up-and-down motion. Try moving just your forehead.

    Allow your breath to adjust itself.

    Start with 1 minute, and build to 8 to 9 minutes.

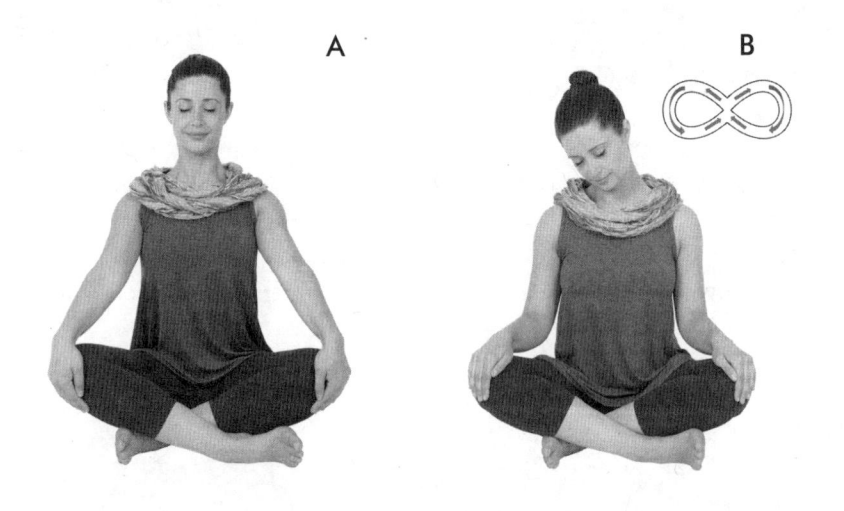

2. Remain in Easy Pose, with your hands on your knees.

    (B) Begin to roll the neck in a sideways figure 8 (∞).

    The chin should come down to the center of the chest twice to complete the full movement.

    The timing is equal for each side of the movement.

Start with 1 minute, and build to 3 minutes.

To finish, be still for 30 seconds, with the head up and neck straight.

3.   (C) Bring your arms straight out to the sides at shoulder level, parallel to the ground, hands in fists, thumbs outside.

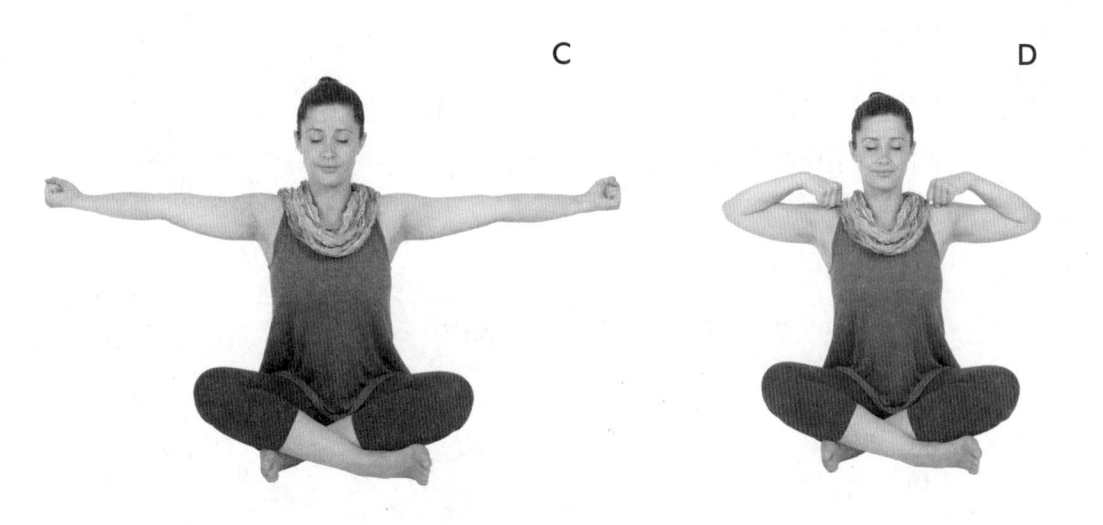

(D) Inhale and bring both fists to the tops of your shoulders while stretching the elbows out as powerfully as possible (flexing your biceps as well).

Return to the original position with arms extended on the exhale.

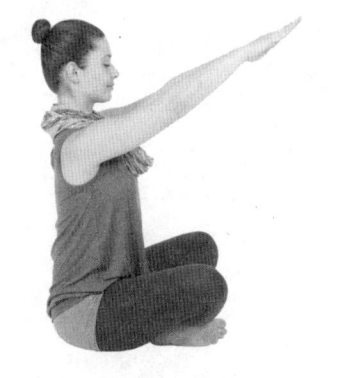

Begin with 1 minute; you can build to 9 minutes.

4.   (E) Stretch your arms out in front at a 45-degree angle, with the fingers pressed together and the palms facing down.

Begin moving the head comfortably in a side-to-side motion for 20 seconds (you can build to 1 minute) as if shaking your head no.

Inhale and suspend the breath briefly. Exhale and relax the breath, relax the posture.

Follow this yoga set with Long Deep Breathing for one to three minutes. Then try the One-Minute Breath, which is a balanced, symmetrical breath that helps improve your psychological state and respiratory self-control. It also helps you focus on three elements of breathing: the inhalation, the pausing to hold the breath, and the exhalation. This breath is said to improve cooperation between both hemispheres of the brain and to create openess to the present moment.

KY MEDITATION:
One-Minute Breath

(Bhajan 2003, 91)

Sit in Easy Pose with your hands in gyan mudra.

Close your eyes and focus at the point between your eyebrows.

Inhale for 5 seconds (build to 20 seconds).

Hold for 5 seconds (build to 20 seconds).

Exhale for 5 seconds (build to 20 seconds).

Repeat and continue the breathing sequence.

Begin with 1 minute; you can build to 11 minutes.

Inhale and suspend the breath briefly. Exhale and relax the breath, relax the posture.

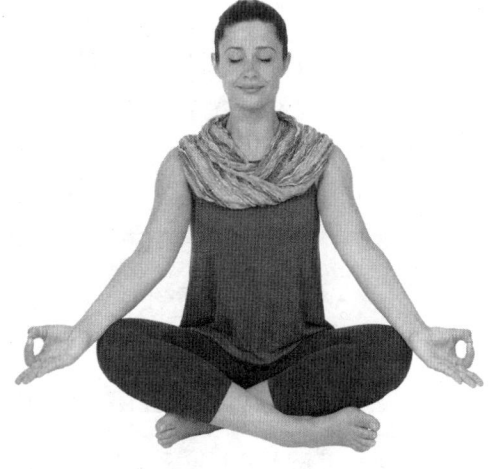

To remember: The segments of this breath are equal. If you're unable to start with 5 seconds, then begin with less, remembering to keep the segments the same duration of time.

When you finish the One-Minute Breath meditation, take a moment and allow your breathing to return to normal.

In Summary

Because the mind and body are fluidly connected, we have shared techniques in this chapter to quiet your body *and* regulate your breath to address anxiety and panic. As you start to recognize the connection between your mind and your body—how one, without fail, affects the other—you will recognize how this relationship works physiologically and cognitively in your own body and mind. When you know *how* to quiet and calm both your body and your mind, you have a very powerful tool to address anxiety and panic. Your daily practice this week will help you experience this connection, use it to manage anxiety and panic, and reduce the frequency of their occurrence.

Week 2 Daily Y-CBT Practice

Guiding Principle

The mind and body are fluidly connected. The state of one is dependent on the state of the other. As one shifts, the other will follow in kind.

Yoga and Meditation

1. Set for Clear Thinking

2. Long Deep Breathing

3. If you have panic attacks, practice the Antidote Breath and Silent Listening Within

Daily Living Practice

This week you will learn about anxiety and panic, and how they manifest in the body and mind. Understanding what's happening in both areas will help you recognize anxiety and panic when they occur. Take note and practice regular check-ins with yourself throughout the day to become aware of what is going on in your mind and body.

This week, try these techniques several times a day:

*   Become aware of how anxiety affects your mind and body differently, and use the skills taught in this chapter to achieve a state of calm in both.

*   Attend to your anxious thought patterns. Notice how they are related to the tension in your body and your breathing patterns.

*   Become aware of your breathing patterns, and correct them using Natural Breathing to calm your body.

Daily Practice Log

	Sunday		Monday		Tuesday		Wednesday		Thursday		Friday		Saturday	
Time of Day														
	B	A	B	A	B	A	B	A	B	A	B	A	B	A
Yoga/Meditation I Used														
Y-CBT Techniques I Used														

B = Before, A = After

1	2	3	4	5	6	7	8	9	10

Low Anxiety   Moderate Anxiety   High Anxiety

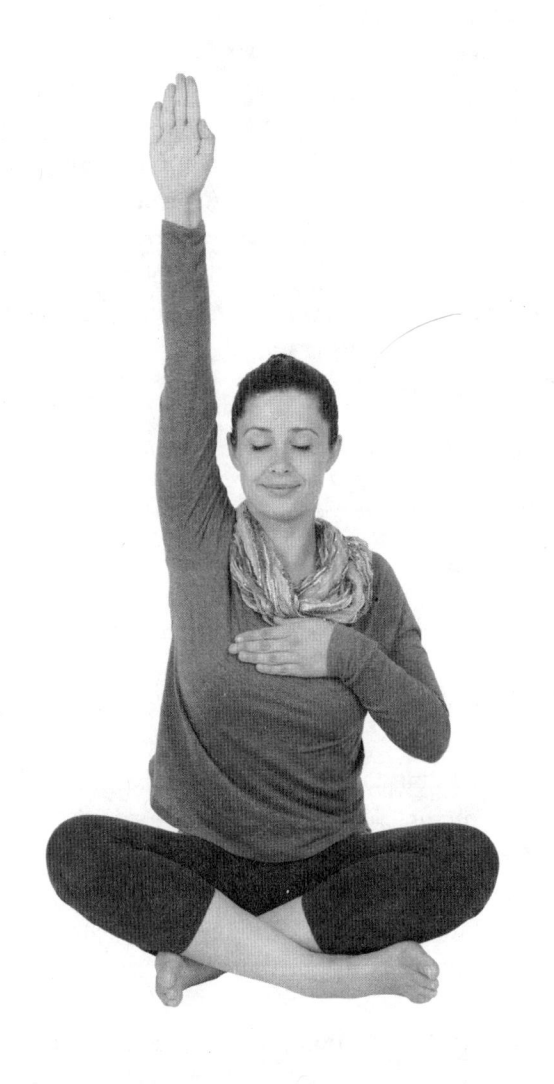

WEEK 3

Working with Worry

When worry consumes us, it can effectively block out everything else in our world. And like so many aspects of anxiety, worry is a cyclical process: it affects our physical state, and that in turn feeds our patterns of worry.

Worry is the primary cognitive feature of anxiety, and it tends to be driven by fear-fueled fantasy in which the facts are lost. Therefore, freedom from worry and anxiety can often be found by focusing on the facts of the situation rather than on a fragmented understanding or fantasy-driven fear. This concept is reflected in this week's guiding principle: *Relief can be found in facts.*

Worry is a funny thing because it fools us into believing that we are doing something productive about a problem or a situation that we likely have no control over. It creates the *illusion* that we are accomplishing something because of all the energy we are expending, but in fact we are doing nothing but filling our minds and bodies with mounting stress.

Can you relate to any of these statements?

I think about the same thing for hours and never get anywhere.

Sometimes I find myself going over a conversation that I had two years ago.

Once I start worrying, I can't stop. It's almost automatic.

Worrying is one of the most common human responses to stress. Everybody worries at some point. But given that worry is so futile, why do we keep doing it?

First, let's define the term. *Worry* is your mind's attempt to remain actively engaged in a problem that is most likely in the past or the future—and therefore out of your control.

When you worry, your mind is busy, and so your body becomes activated and energized. This active state makes you *feel* as if you are doing something constructive. For example, let's say you are throwing a party next weekend. As the date gets closer, every night you lie in bed and begin to think about the food: what if it's not ready on time, or there isn't enough, or no one likes it? You think about the space: cleaning it, decorating it, moving things around. What if something goes wrong? What if it rains? What if no one comes? This swirl in your thoughts keeps you very busy when you should be sleeping.

Lying in bed worrying doesn't get the food prepared, or the space decorated, so the process is simply exhausting and futile. The more you worry, the more tense and fatigued your body feels. In the moment, all of this anticipatory anxiety keeps you actively engaged in your fears, which makes you *feel* as if you are in control of them. However, there is nothing actually being accomplished. As noted above, no matter how much energy you expend on worry, it accomplishes nothing other than putting you into this futile activated state, which only leaves you feeling exhausted.

Worry should not be confused with logical problem solving. The difference is that worry actually *constricts* our thinking rather than opening it up to possible solutions. Instead of moving toward productive outcomes and the resolution of a problem, worry just keeps us going around in circles.

The next time you are lying in bed worrying about something, get up, turn on the light, and make an organized list of the things you need to do and when you will do them. Take note of the things that are outside of your control—the weather or other people's behavior, for instance—and do your best to let those go.

Understanding the process of worry, and how to move beyond it to more productive thought patterns, is essential in managing anxiety and stress.

Three Aspects of Worry

Because worry creates the illusion that you have more control than you actually do, that busy, active feeling can be strangely comforting. That is one reason it's so seductive.

Typically, there are three aspects to worry: reviewing the problem, attempting to predict the future with negative outcomes, and ultimately creating a series of illogical or impractical solutions in an attempt to solve a problem that, in most cases, is outside of your control.

Reviewing the Problem

Reviewing the problem, or ruminating about it, is central to the worrying process. When you worry, you remain actively engaged with the problem by rehashing the details. This will often involve a continual replay in the mind of what was said or an intense review of what was done.

By re-creating and replaying such details, you remain engaged in the problem and succumb to the illusion that the focus of the worry is still *in play*. It's as if this process effectively *suspends time*, as you remain caught up in the affective, or emotional, components of the worrisome situation. Simply put, when you worry about something in the past, you are emotionally reliving the moment of stress.

Let's consider Michael, who had a conversation with his boss about work performance. Ever since the conversation, Michael has been replaying the event in his mind. He has been mulling over every word said, over and over, so much that they've taken on grander proportions. What was in reality a constructive conversation has become, in Michael's mind, a heated argument that has put Michael on the defensive. As he relives the conversation word for word, he begins to believe that he said the wrong thing, or that he should've said a different thing—that his boss is out to get him because the boss had negative comments about Michael's work performance. He can't stop worrying about what was said, and his head is throbbing. His breath is shallow, and he feels clammy and sweaty.

Laura, on the other hand, can't stop worrying about the exam she took. Ever since she finished, she's been reviewing the questions and answers in her mind, over and over, wondering which she got right or wrong. As she replays the details of the exam she loses track of how she answered: Had she selected A or D? Which one really is correct? She begins to think the exam was filled with trick questions, and that maybe none of her answers were right. She can't end her fears about what happened and can't concentrate on anything else. Her neck and shoulders are tense, and she feels light-headed from unconsciously holding her breath.

Like Michael and Laura, if you suffer from severe bouts of worry, it's often the case that you can't stop thinking about what happened. Right? The scenario plays over and over again in your mind, but this repetition brings you no reprieve from the pain and can even add to your anxiety. Maintaining this level of engagement in the moment of stress offers a counterintuitive but oddly effective sense of relief, because you're still fully involved in the past event.

The emotional experience goes something like this: *If I am reliving these events, they are in my present rather than my past.* If these events are allowed to fall into the worrier's past, then they become unchangeable. So, as long as the worrier can remain in this state of reviewing and repeating, the events causing the concern are still in the *affective* or *emotional present* and, therefore, suspended in time. This offers the irrational prospect that the events of the past are negotiable. This is why Michael imagines that he had said something different to his boss, and why Laura is debating whether she checked answer B rather than C. They are attempting to manipulate a past event in order to feel better—but the opposite happens and they just go around in circles or the situation just becomes direr!

Of course, the past is not negotiable. What happened in the past is past, and we can't change it. What Michael doesn't know yet is that accepting what *actually* happened and moving forward from there is how he can find genuine relief.

Predicting the Future with Negative Outcomes

When you struggle with worry, you may find that when confronted with the facts of the past the quality of the worry begins to change, and you might experience a shift in your thinking process. When you begin to accept the true details of what happened, the focus of the fear can shift to the future. Instead of moving forward in a productive way, you begin to imagine worst-case outcomes.

Michael's exaggerated thoughts have left him feeling completely humiliated. He's sure that he won't get the promotion he asked for, that he won't get the raise he was counting on. Now he's convinced that his boss will fire him. Laura has convinced herself that she failed the exam, which means she'll fail the course, which means she'll never get a job.

During this type of worry, as with Michael and Laura, you have the desire to gain control over a situation that feels out of control. Only this time you try to predict what could happen at a later date. You might engage in aftermath and anticipatory anxious thought. You might conjure up every possible future scenario! In a strange way, imagining the worst actually offers you a solution and, thus, an *illusion* of control. When caught up in this process, it can feel like predicting and planning for the most exaggerated worst-case outcome is better than waiting for the unknown, future events to happen. This upside-down sense of control—the pivotal feature here—provides some relief from the intense worry and fear of the unknown.

Such worrying can take on extreme proportions. Worriers can quickly imagine themselves as homeless, jobless, friendless, or penniless when, in fact, these fantasies usually bear no relation to reality. These thought processes are in most cases simply a self-defeating coping mechanism—an attempt to "prepare for" an onslaught of negative events that the mind has fabricated in response to worry.

Creating Illogical Solutions

As you face the reality of events and the possibility of extreme negative outcomes, your mind begins to barter. This process is the most illogical and problematic of all. The worrying might go on for hours, perhaps days. All events have been reviewed; all negative outcomes have been delineated. All that is left for you to do is to create "solutions." The "solutions," built on the worry and the conclusions drawn, are often extreme, illogical, and sometimes harmfully life changing.

We all search for solutions when we have problems. But this kind of intense worry often causes us to create illogical or even irrational plans in an attempt to come to a premature resolution of the problem. You may be desperate for the rumination to stop, and it can feel like the only way to do this is to come up with a solution. Because fear is driving the process and blowing the problem out of proportion, the facts of the situation are lost or distorted. And so, illogical solutions created by the worrying mind will often take on a fatalistic bent.

The process of worry replaces logic in Laura's case too. Her "solution" is that she will drop of out of school. Since she's going to fail the course anyway, better to just leave school and forget about all higher education. Michael's "solution" is to sell his house. He's going to lose his job, he won't have an income, and he'll be too humiliated to look for work elsewhere. It's time to put his house on the market.

Whether your worry takes the form of reviewing the past or trying to predict the future, you have probably found yourself creating illogical solutions to end the worry cycle. *Reviewing the past* and *predicting the future* offer you a false sense of control over the uncontrollable. Remaining engaged or ruminating over the events of the past is futile, and attempting to predict the future is impossible—especially when the vision is fueled by fear. In order to get to a different place, it is important to remember that worry is a funny thing because it fools you into thinking you are doing something about a situation that you can't control. That's because your mind and body are engaged. But the truth is, that agitated process accomplishes the opposite of what you are hoping for. It keeps you stuck and anxious, and sometimes causes you to make decisions that are self-defeating or even harmful.

EXERCISE:
Identify Your Worry Patterns

Understanding your worry patterns is helpful because you can learn to catch yourself in the process and change the direction in which your mind is moving. Use this exercise to familiarize yourself with your worry patterns.

1. When I worry, I review the problem over and over again: yes _____ no _____

    List examples of the types of situations that you tend to worry about by reviewing the details of what happened over and over again.

    Example: *An upsetting conversation with my boss*

    _____

    _____

    _____

    Write down an example of the dialogue in your head when you are reviewing the problem:

    _____

    _____

    _____

2. When I worry, I predict the future with negative outcomes: yes _____ no _____

    List some examples of the types of situations that lead you to attempt to predict the future.

    Example: *I talked too much at the meeting; I know everyone will be mad at me this afternoon.*

    _____

    _____

    _____

Write down an example of the dialogue in your head when you are predicting the future:

_____

_____

_____

3. When I worry, I create illogical solutions: yes _____ no _____

List some situations in which you have created an illogical solution to your worry.

Example: *I decided to send an e-mail out to apologize to everyone who was at the meeting. No one knew what I was talking about. I was really embarrassed.*

Write down an example of the dialogue in your head when you are trying to come up with solutions to your worry:

_____

_____

_____

Now that you have an understanding of your worry patterns, it's time to examine your often-automatic mind-body patterns of worry. You'll also learn valuable techniques to help you address these patterns and thus break the worry cycle.

Breaking the Worry Cycle

You can learn to quiet your mind and your body simultaneously, and thereby successfully disrupt the cycle of worry. This process is more than just a thinking problem, and simply changing the direction of your thoughts won't do the trick, because the anxious state of your body will trigger more rumination and racing thoughts. If you can achieve a relaxed state in both your mind and your body, you will be able to develop solutions from a more logical, fact-based perspective.

When you find your thoughts running from point A to point B and back again without establishing any conclusion or logical plan, the following meditation, Powering Down to Transform Anxiety, can help. When you are anxious, your body is tense and agitated, and at the same time your mind is racing with a swirl of worry that feels insurmountable. Each will instantaneously trigger the other, creating that unpleasant, uncomfortable cycle of anxiety. Powering down through meditation will help you train yourself to respond to stressful situations with a relaxed physical state and a focus on factual information. Focusing on the facts will almost always quiet undefined fear and allow you to move forward with more productive problem solving.

MEDITATION:
Powering Down to Transform Anxiety

This meditation is designed to progressively quiet your body by regulating your breath and releasing tension while *at the same time* relaxing your mind by focusing on factual information. When you focus on any simple fact, the process of worry or rumination will be disabled in your thought process, and rational problem solving can emerge.

As with other meditations that are new to you, practice this several times when you are *not* worrying to build familiarity and ease with the process. When you do find yourself starting to worry, you will have this powerful calming tool at the ready.

1. First, choose a comfortable seat, preferably with a solid back. Close your eyes and become aware of your breath.

2. Next, take note that your mind is spinning, and be aware of the tension in your body.

3. Shift your posture by positioning your feet firmly on the ground, your hands on the arms of the chair or on your knees, your back pressed squarely against the back of the chair, and your seat resting evenly in the seat of the chair.

4. Take a deep breath in, and as you exhale, physically push or drop your shoulders down. You will notice that your elbows and wrists will also shift. Release the tension in these joints too. Repeat.

5. Take a deep breath in, and on the exhale direct your attention to the soles of your feet and where and how they meet the floor. Repeat.

6. Take a deep breath in, and on the exhale direct your attention to the place where your seat meets the seat, and allow yourself to sink comfortably and deeply into the chair. You will notice that other parts of your body will relax too. Repeat.

7. Take a deep breath in, and on the exhale direct your attention to the place where the small of your back meets the back of the chair. Consider the image of a cat curled up in the corner of a sofa, safe and protected. Repeat.

8. Take a deep breath in, and on the exhale, with your eyes remaining closed, focus on the place between your eyebrows at the bridge of your nose. For a moment, attend to what you "see" there. It might be lights or swirls of color.

9. Next, consider *one* fact. Choose a simple indisputable fact, one that is impossible to argue: *Water is wet. The sky is blue. I like peppermint.* Imagine this fact "sitting" at the space between your eyebrows at the bridge of your nose. And breathe deeply as you repeat this fact silently to yourself.

10. Take a deep breath in, and on the exhale focus on the following things in a smooth and rhythmic way:

    • The fact

    • Your shoulders down

    • The small of your back

    • Where your seat meets the seat

    • The soles of your feet

    Repeat.

11. Observe your experience of simultaneously having a calm, quietly engaged mind and a calm, relaxed physical experience. Continue this for three minutes.

Relief Can Be Found in Facts

As noted earlier, worry makes you feel as if you are actively engaged with an event that is in the past or the future, giving you the illusion that you have control over events that are, in fact, outside of your control. Expending energy on reviewing and sometimes "rewriting" history, or predicting the future and creating illogical solutions, only deepens your problems. These are usually ill-fated coping strategies. It is important to remind yourself that you cannot change the past and you cannot predict the future.

Worry begets anxiety, which creates feelings that constrict you both physically and emotionally. When you learn to quiet the physical symptoms of anxiety, you will find that the constant pulse of negative thinking is naturally reduced. A quieter mind and a calmer physical state allow the mind to be directed to a more logical and fact-based discussion of the problem. Words like "never" and "always" rarely apply to a fact-based analysis of a problem. Problems become solvable when they are framed as identifiable, well-defined dilemmas with attainable courses of action.

EXERCISE:
Quieting the Mind and the Body with Facts

This exercise is designed to help you begin to move away from worry and focus more productively on the facts of the situation.

1. When you are caught in a cycle of worry, stay focused on the facts of the situation. The facts are the facts. You cannot change them. Consider a situation that you have been worrying about. It may be a conversation that you had or a task that you are concerned about completing. Write it below.

    Example: *I told two different people that I would help them next weekend with a project. I keep going over it and over it in my head. I can't do both, and someone will be angry with me if I cancel.*

    _____

    _____

    _____

2. Sit in a quiet place. Spend several minutes practicing Long Deep Breathing (see Week 2). Scan the physical state of your body. Notice your heart rate. Notice where you feel tension. Listen to your breath. Allow your breath to be your focus. Try to keep your mind clear. Focus on a neutral object or thought, such as a smooth stone or running water, or a simple, indisputable fact.

3. When your mind is in a calm and neutral state, slowly return to the situation you are worrying about. Consider the facts of the situation. If your mind begins to focus on what could happen, gently shift your attention back to the facts. List all of the facts, no matter how minor.

Example: *I promised Tina I would help her move some boxes to storage next weekend. Tina has an injured shoulder. She has a small car, I have a truck. I also promised Jose I would help him plan out a vegetable garden. I have experience with gardens, he does not. There are two days in a weekend. I also have to take my dog to the vet next weekend.*

_____

_____

_____

4. With your facts in mind, slowly try to review realistic options. List reasonable actions you might take that are based in the facts of the situation.

   Example: *I can ask Tina if she can wait another week, when I have more time. I can ask Jose if he can delay another week. I can honestly explain the situation to both people— they may offer a solution that also works in my favor. I am a responsible person and rarely have to cancel. I can be kind to myself and realize that I can only do so much.*

_____

_____

_____

5. What information or other factors do you still need to consider in order to devise a realistic plan?

   Example: *I need to recognize that my needs are just as important as my friends' needs. While my goal is to be helpful to others, I need to realistically consider how much I can do. I have to consider that others won't automatically be angry with me if I am honest. I need to remember that I can say no to projects and still be a good friend.*

_____

_____

_____

6. Resume Long Deep Breathing. Has your heart rate changed? Can you hear your breath? Is your mind focused on a neutral object or thought?

7. Create a plan: based on the facts that you have written and the options that you have pondered, create a logical, step-by-step plan to manage the problem.

    Example: *I will call Tina and explain that while I would like to help her this weekend, I need to delay until next weekend.*

    _____

    _____

    _____

The solution to your problem might not be clear immediately, and that's okay. Sometimes it simply takes a while to work things out. You may need to acquire more information before you can create a plan. You may need to simply accept the situation and do nothing for the moment. And sometimes, there is nothing that you can do to change your circumstances. The goal is to learn to stay calm when you have a problem to solve and do the best you can to work through it. Worry and rumination will not help you with that.

The impulse to predict negative outcomes and create illogical solutions can be strong and seemingly inescapable. The good news is that you can learn to reduce these urges and, over time, get rid of them. The process to do so is what you'll learn next.

Acknowledge, Comfort, Calm, and Inspire

If you are having a hard time quieting your thoughts and your physical responses, you are not alone. Sometimes it's just a matter of organizing your approach, which can be done in four basic steps. First, you will learn to become aware of and acknowledge your emotional state and its *sensory signature*. This is your personal physical response to stress. Next, you will learn how to quiet or comfort yourself during anxious moments with *reassurance*. Then you'll discover how to use *yogic movement* to calm your body and mind. Finally, you will be encouraged to find *inspiration* from enduring wisdom to help you tackle problems from an uplifted perspective.

Step 1: Acknowledge Your Sensory Signature of Worry

As you now know, when we worry, we often generate negative outcomes and create illogical solutions. We may even get mad at ourselves for worrying and try to push the thoughts away, telling ourselves, "Oh, stop worrying! You're crazy!"

Instead of engaging in this kind of self-critical thinking, you can learn how to mindfully observe and acknowledge how you feel by actively engaging your attention and noticing what's going on in your mind and body.

All people have a unique set of thoughts and bodily sensations that consistently convey the experience of worry to them. We call this unique pattern the *sensory signature of worry*. It comprises the thoughts you repeat to yourself and the very small physical movements your body makes, called *micromovements*, that together equal the experience of worry for you. An example of a sensory signature might be: "I know I'm worried because I feel scared, my stomach is tight, and I am repeating, over and over again, *What will I do if something bad happens today?*"

How do *you* think and feel when you experience worry? Ask yourself, "How do I know I'm worried?" Take a moment to consider what goes on in your thoughts, breath, and body. Are you reviewing the past, predicting negative outcomes, or creating reactive solutions? How is your breathing? Where is the worry located in your body? Do you try to push away thoughts or get angry with yourself for being anxious?

Here is an example of the elements that make up the sensory signature of worry:

Breath: "I can hardly breathe."

Thought: "I said the wrong thing!"

Body: "I feel so shaky, and my shoulders are so tight!"

It's not always easy to identify your thoughts and what is going on with your breathing and in your body when you are in the process of worrying. The following exercise will help you understand your typical mental and physical states when you are experiencing the distress of worry.

EXERCISE:
Identify Your Sensory Signature of Worry

Answer the following questions to better pinpoint what happens in your own body and mind when you begin to worry.

1. What am I thinking? Am I worried about the past or predicting something negative about the future?

    _____

    _____

    _____

2. How am I breathing? Is my breath fast or slow? Deep or shallow?

    _____

    _____

    _____

3. How do I experience worry in my body?

    What is my posture like? _____

    How do my neck and my shoulders feel? _____

    How does my stomach feel? _____

    Am I moving my foot rapidly? _____

    Am I looking down, trying not to make eye contact? _____

    Other: _____

The goal of acknowledging your sensory signature of worry at this stage is to simply learn to become aware of your total mind-body experience and accept that state as it is. Acknowledging and accepting how you feel allows you to begin the next step, which is using comfort and self-compassion to quiet and shift your physical and mental states.

Step 2: Comfort Yourself

Once you identify your mental and physical patterns of response, you can begin to transform the way you experience worry and anxiety in general. You can relax your tight chest, deepen your breathing, and replace negative images with positive ones. You can also learn to comfort yourself. (In a sense, you are acting as your own coach.) For instance, you can change your thinking to "It's okay. I can relax my stomach and breathe into it. Maybe things will turn out okay. The truth is, I can't really predict the future anyway."

All of us want to be acknowledged and accepted by others, and it is just as important to accept yourself. Often, we try to comfort ourselves with nice words, but that doesn't work on its own, because our bodies are still tense. You need to acknowledge your worry, comfort yourself, *and* relax your body. Use the exercise below to practice this process.

EXERCISE:
Practicing Self-Comfort

Here are three ways you can practice self-comfort. Read each supportive statement a few times and then answer the questions.

1. *Breath:* I notice that my breath is shallow or rapid. I can attend to this issue and comfort myself by relaxing and deepening my breath (see Natural Breathing, Week 2).

   Am I breathing through my mouth or my nose? _____

   Is my chest rising when I inhale and receding on the exhale? _____

   Is my stomach expanding with each inhale? _____

2. *Thoughts:* Once I become aware that I have started worrying, instead of feeding my worry with self-criticism, picturing negative outcomes, or creating unrealistic solutions, I can use my deepened breath to accept how I feel and comfort myself with these statements:

   I am aware that I'm afraid. It's okay to be afraid. In this situation, anyone would be.

   I'm aware that I feel really upset. I'll get through this. This feeling will pass if I am kind to myself.

My kind self-talk to quiet my thoughts:

_____

_____

_____

3. *Body:* Once I recognize that parts of my body are tight, I can use my breath and my words to relax them.

Example: *I am noticing that my stomach is clenched. I'll gently ask myself to shift my attention to my breath and breathe into my stomach to comfort and relax it. My shoulders and chest feel very tight. I'll breathe into them deeply and kindly say to myself, "It's okay. I'll do better if I relax. I can relax my shoulders."*

My kind self-talk to quiet my body:

_____

_____

_____

Practicing self-comfort involves first acknowledging and accepting how you feel so that you are more receptive to the comfort that follows. However, when you are anxious, your body may still be stressed. To feel fully comforted, then, you need to calm your body as well. The next step accomplishes this goal.

Step 3: Calm Yourself with Movement

Words of acknowledgment and comfort can help, but sometimes they are not enough on their own, and your body may need additional help. If you are still worried or anxious after step 2, the next step is to do some movement and meditation to help restructure your mind-body pattern. You may choose to do one or both of these simple yogic movements.

These movements will help you shed anxious physical energy so you can more easily calm yourself and better manage anxious feelings. Studies have shown that physical activities such as walking and other exercise can be very helpful in reducing anxiety (Streeter et al. 2010). This may be because exercise can relax tight muscle patterns, deepen breathing, and replace stressful hormonal patterns with more calming hormones (Dusek and Benson 2009).

When you finish the following yoga sets, you'll notice yourself breathing differently, and perhaps you'll feel new sensations. Your body might be tingly, or you might feel a little light-headed. That's okay—it is part of the adjustment your body is making as you learn to move and breathe in new ways. As long as you maintain the new breathing, you're likely to find your mind less worried as well

YOGA:
Release Anxiety

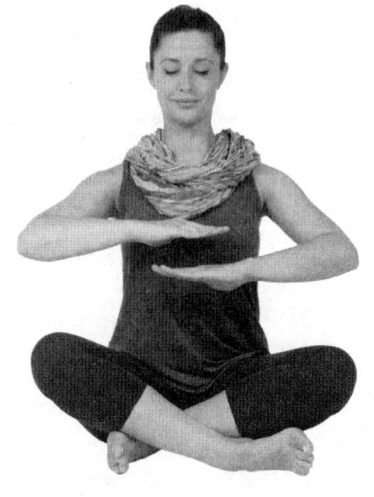

Give your physical body something constructive to do when it's showing symptoms of anxiety or worry. This exercise will channel energy in a positive direction.

1. Sit comfortably in a chair or in Easy Pose on the floor.

2. Stack your flat hands on top of each other, leaving 3 to 4 inches of space between. Then move the top hand away from you and then begin to roll one hand around the other, making a circling motion.

3. Keep up this motion for 1 minute.

4. Inhale deeply, hold, then exhale.

YOGA:
Let Go of Anxiety

Release more tense energy with this exercise, which ends with a calming breath pattern.

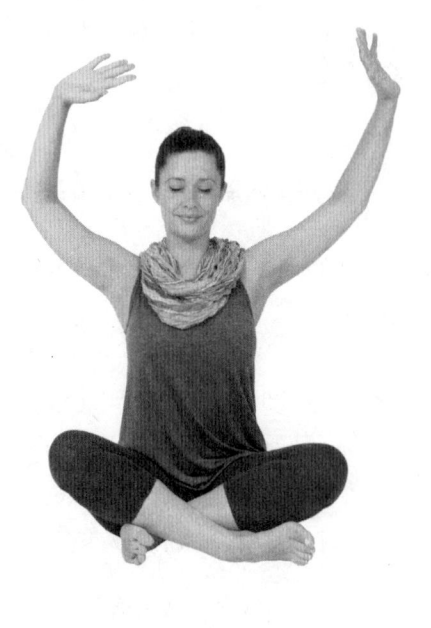

1. Sit comfortably in a chair or in Easy Pose on the floor.

2. Raise your arms up above your shoulders, fingers spread.

3. Shake your hands, then shake your arms, then shake your shoulders, and then shake your whole body. Even your legs and feet can move. Continue for 30 seconds.

4. When you finish, relax your arms and sit up straight.

Inhale and suspend the breath briefly. Exhale and relax the breath, relax the posture.

When you are finshed, practice Long Deep Breathing for 2 minutes (see Week 2 for instructions).

Step 4: Find Inspiration

Wisdom can be a powerful medicine. Reading the thoughts of sagacious women and men can help us shift toward a more positive and spirited outlook. It can inspire us to become our best selves and accomplish even the most difficult goals. Wisdom can also uplift us, giving us strength to face our anxious moments.

Having confidence and believing in oneself can also do wonders. The belief that we *can* do something seems to be at once energizing and relaxing.

The following Victory Meditation can help you develop a new belief system about your abilities. Struggling with anxiety can create an expectation of defeat. The Victory Meditation offers you a metaphor for building within you an expectation of victory *instead of* defeat. This exercise is not meant to be strenuous. Rather, the goal is to physically change your emotional reflex from "giving up" when stressed to believing that you can be victorious. The word "victory" can serve as a personal affirmation when you are feeling anxious. The affirmation and "to remember" text in this meditation are quoted from Yogi Bhajan.

KY MEDITATION:
Victory Meditation

(Bhajan 1992)

Sit in Easy Pose.

Raise your right arm straight up from the shoulder, perpendicular to the ground, the palm facing forward.

Place your left hand on the heart center, with the elbow relaxed at the side.

Close your eyes.

Inhale, hold, and exhale. Breathe consciously. Make your breath the longest, strongest, most conscious self-controlled breath that you can.

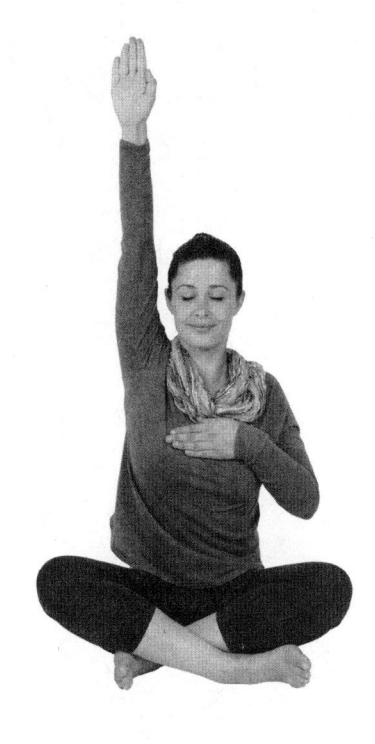

Make an affirmation: Silently repeat the word "victory" as many times as you can. "Engrave it in every molecule. Just learn this one word. When you feel like putting your hand down, stretch it higher— that is the victory!"

Begin with 1 to 2 minutes, and build to 6 to 7 minutes.

To end: Inhale deeply, hold tightly, and stretch the body for 20 seconds. Then exhale and relax.

Inhale and suspend the breath briefly. Exhale and relax the breath, relax the posture.

To remember: "Victory is my goal; victory is my strength, victory is my guide; victory is my teacher… Victory. It's a very powerful word."

Not everyone can stretch his or her arm up to 90 degrees straight overhead. That's fine. If your arm begins to fall, you can try to lift it up again, stretch higher, and experience a victory instead of a defeat.

You can use your core muscles with your conscious breath—rather than your arms, upper back, or shoulder muscles—to help you hold the position. Resisting the natural urge to let your arm drop when it tires, and instead raising it higher, offers an empowering experience of triumph rather than defeat.

You can also experience a feeling of victory through the wise words of other people. Below is an exercise for using the wisdom of others to find inspiration.

EXERCISE:
Finding Inspiration

Here is a short list of quotations that have been inspiring to us and our clients. Feel free to add examples that inspire you.

Love is the miracle cure. Loving ourselves works miracles in our lives.—Louise Hay (2004, 17)

Deep at the center of my being, there is an infinite well of love… The more love I use and give, the more I have to give. The supply is endless.—Louise Hay (2004, 102)

Life is a flow of love. Only your participation is requested.—Yogi Bhajan (1985)

Nobody can control anybody. All you can do [is] flow with each other like rivers and streams flow with each other and…end up in the same ocean.—Yogi Bhajan (1983b)

Every thought you have has an energy that will either strengthen or weaken you.—Wayne Dyer (2004b, 71)

Change the way you look at things, and the things you look at change.—Wayne Dyer (2004b, 126)

Add your own inspiring quotations here: _____

_____

_____

Choose one (or more) of the quotations above and write it on an index card, carry it in your pocket, and read it often. When you read the quotation, breathe deeply and imagine that you are breathing in the meaning of the statement, as if you could infuse it in your mind and body.

In Summary

Because worry is a common problem for people who are anxious, we have shared with you a variety of techniques that can help break the worry cycle. As you learn to identify your own worry patterns and practice the techniques in this chapter to quiet your mind and power down, you will gain new skills to combat anxiety. Remember that *relief can be found in facts*. Quieting your mind with facts and logic will help bring the cognitive aspects of anxiety under control. As you become adept at acknowledging, comforting, calming, and inspiring yourself, you'll find yourself taking on a bright new attitude. Over time, you'll find that you are worrying for shorter periods of time and not as often.

Week 3 Daily Y-CBT Practice

Guiding Principle

Relief can be found in facts. Freedom from worry and anxiety can often begin by focusing on the facts or the total truth of the situation rather than on a fragmented understanding or fantasy-driven fear.

Yoga and Meditation

1. Yoga to Release Anxiety

2. Yoga to Let Go of Anxiety

3. Victory Meditation

Daily Living Practice

Your practice this week is to deepen your awareness of what happens in your mind and your body when you are anxious, and to work on quieting your patterns of worry. As you go through each day this week, remind yourself to:

- Notice your worry patterns and begin to change them by challenging the fear with facts.

- Practice Powering Down to Transform Anxiety to experience the state of having a quiet mind and a quiet body.

- Comfort yourself, and challenge yourself to be victorious as you face small and large stresses throughout the week.

- Read the inspirational quote you have written on the index card.

Daily Practice Log

	Sunday		Monday		Tuesday		Wednesday		Thursday		Friday		Saturday	
Time of Day														
	B	A	B	A	B	A	B	A	B	A	B	A	B	A
Yoga/Meditation I Used														
Y-CBT Techniques I Used														

B = Before, A = After

1	2	3	4	5	6	7	8	9	10
Low Anxiety				Moderate Anxiety				High Anxiety	

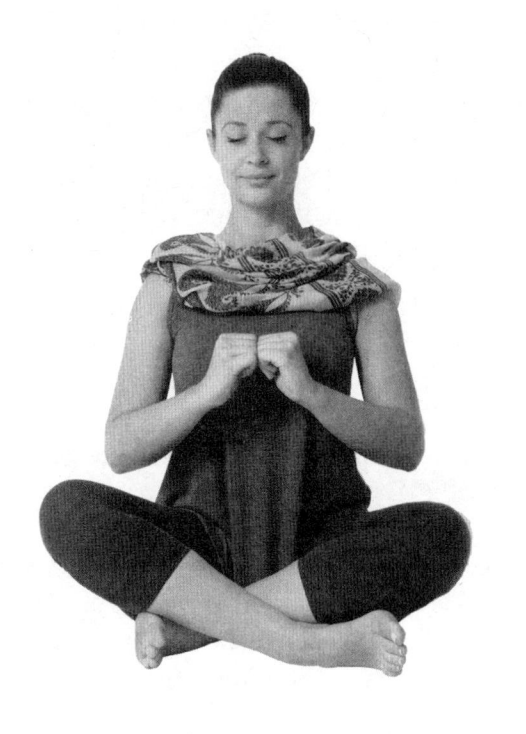

WEEK 4

Finding Your Value

Anxiety can often cause us to lose perspective on our strengths and all that we have to offer. In fact, every one of us possesses profound and unique value. The material in this chapter can help you reclaim or redefine your finest attributes. Or, if you have never connected with these positive personal attributes, it will provide an opportunity to discover them for the first time.

As you move through this chapter, we ask you to consider this guiding principle: **Habits of the mind influence our lives.** What you think affects how you feel. Your thoughts are of your own making. Because you are the only one who is thinking your thoughts, you can choose to create habits of the mind that claim your self-value and give you freedom from anxiety.

In this chapter, we look at the factors that contribute to each person's overall sense of worth. First, we will introduce the concept of *intrinsic value*, which holds that all people have innate worth that is unchanging, regardless of the challenges they face in life. The second concept speaks to the importance of identifying and strengthening a set of core inspirational principles that guide us in our life choices—what we call an *internal guidance system* (IGS). This chapter will address how these concepts, along with self-compassion, can reduce anxiety and support a greater sense of self-worth.

Discovering Your Intrinsic Value

Intrinsic value is a term that we have borrowed from the world of finance. This phrase describes the essential, inherent value of something, such as a currency, that persists regardless of the current market value.

In Y-CBT, we apply this concept to self-worth and the building of self-esteem. In this context, intrinsic value refers to every person's cluster of positive personal attributes that remain true regardless of what is happening around or to that individual. These positive qualities remain intact within each of us and are *intrinsically* present, even when we are caught up in the difficult swirl of life and relationships.

Regardless of what life puts in your path, your value is constant and unchanging. Bad things happen all the time, to everyone, but these things do not define us. Our value remains intact even when we are struggling in difficult times.

The same principle applies to the way you are treated by others. Measuring your value by the behavior of others leaves you vulnerable. Too often, people look for their worth to be reflected by the words or actions of other people. For instance, if you receive a compliment, you may believe that you are worthy; if you receive a criticism, you think that you are worthless. The fact is, whether a person treats you well or poorly, the behavior of the other person is *not* a reflection of your value. That person's behavior is a reflection of who *he* or *she* is, not who *you* are. It is your challenge to define and acknowledge your own sense of value in the world and discover what you believe to be true about yourself.

As you consider this concept, you may find yourself developing an argument either about yourself or the human condition in general. You might be thinking, "But I really am stupid! I just can't get a job" or "No one will love me. I'm not worthy of love. Look at all my failed relationships!" You might also be thinking, "What about Hitler? What about serial killers? They have committed unthinkable crimes! How can they have intrinsic value?" Comparing yourself to those who have done heinous deeds is not productive thinking. Yes, evil may exist in the world, but you should not allow that fact to stall your ability to search for and recognize your own value in the world. If you find yourself following this line of thinking in response to this concept, it might be helpful for you to consider why your thoughts go to such extremes to avoid exploring *your* intrinsic value.

Quieting Negative Self-Talk

Again and again we hear all-encompassing, negative self-statements from people who struggle with anxiety. The constant press of anxious thoughts and feelings creates self-doubt that invades and erodes a person's ability to accurately evaluate sense of worth. As a result, people develop false beliefs such as:

I am worthless.

I have terrible luck.

I never do anything right.

Everyone hates me.

I am always wrong.

I am always anxious.

I am a loser.

I am my own worst enemy.

Overarching negative beliefs of this nature can develop for a variety of reasons. You might become self-critical and judgmental following a series of personal challenges that you have faced. Or, if you are in problematic relationships with people who are critical or cruel, you may begin to accept their negative opinions of you. But remember, just because someone expresses his or her opinion, it doesn't make him or her *right*.

Regardless of the cause, we often find that people who struggle with anxiety develop a negative self-definition. This impacts their ability to hold on to a core set of positive self-beliefs that allow them to feel successful, proud, and happy.

Repeating negative statements to yourself will cause you to develop a limited, inaccurate, and negative picture of who you are. Filling your mind with thoughts of your limitations or mistakes leaves no room for you to consider your strengths. A mistake is simply a mistake. You are not defined by it, and it does not change your intrinsic value. No one is always worthless. No one is always anxious. No one is always wrong. No one is always *anything*.

Breaking the mental habit of self-doubt and criticism, and embracing a fluency in your strengths and personal value, require your full attention. Of course you have worth! Everyone does. You are probably even aware of some of your strengths. But managing symptoms of stress and anxiety over a long period of time may have caused you to begin overattending to the negative while ignoring, minimizing, or discounting your positive attributes.

Many of us are hesitant about speaking about our strengths or skills for fear of being seen as bragging or conceited. You are probably even downplaying your talents right now as you read this and are considering what you're good—or not good—at! But acknowledging your strengths does not mean that you are claiming to be perfect or think you have no areas of growth to work on! Learning to acknowledge your value and strengths is how you can begin to build a more balanced and accurate view of yourself.

The following exercise is designed to help you begin to draw out from within yourself an accurate, honest assessment of your positive attributes. Your task in this process is to take an open and authentic look at the strengths you have within you and learn to own them from a place of clarity and acceptance.

EXERCISE:
Identify Your Intrinsic Value

Try this exercise each morning or at the end of the day as part of your daily practice.

Make a list of three positive personal qualities that you possess and that you believe to be true about yourself. These attributes can be large or small. They might be particular qualities, for example, "I am smart, funny, and patient." They might be talents: "I am a good dancer, a good cook, a fast learner." They might describe character strengths, such as being a loving parent, helpful to others, a hard worker.

Begin with just three. As you move through your daily routine, begin to pay attention to your strengths and the things that are valuable about you. Notice what you do well and the things that come easily to you. Perhaps you have come to ignore these attributes. Name and put words to them: "I am creative. I am articulate. I am trustworthy."

Notice the people who care for you and whom you care for. Name and put words to what you bring to these relationships: "I am kind. I am generous. I am dependable."

My intrinsic value:

1. _____

2. _____

3. _____

Each week, add to this list at least two new positive qualities that you observe in yourself and that you believe are intrinsically true about who you are.

Review your list as you begin your daily practice each day. Put these characteristics in the forefront of your mind as you breathe. Become fluent in your intrinsic value by embedding these qualities in your internal portrait of yourself.

Very often we notice positive qualities in others that we ignore or discount in ourselves. The next exercise asks you to take a moment to consider the positive qualities that you recognize in others. This gives you a frame of reference so you are consciously aware of the qualities that you believe admirable people possess.

EXERCISE:
The Good Person

We all have an *ideal persona* that we aspire to live up to. Consider for a moment the qualities that you admire in your own conception of a "good person." Breathe deeply and mindfully as you think about each prompt.

What are the measures of a good person?

List your thoughts:

_____

_____

_____

_____

_____

_____

Next, review the list, and take note of which of these characteristics you possess. Write them down:

_____

_____

_____

Are you surprised that you possess some of the positive characteristics that make up your "good person"? This would not surprise us at all, and it is not a coincidence. When you are struggling with anxious thoughts and self-doubt, some of your strengths may dim in your mind. This exercise offers you the opportunity to remind yourself of the good qualities that you possess but that you may only notice in other people.

As you focus on your own positive qualities, you will begin to understand them as part of your intrinsic value, characteristics that are always true about you. You will find that you can hold on to and rely on these personal attributes when life gets hard.

Shifting from a negative self-view and embracing your intrinsic value will take some time and attention. The following section will teach you how to treat yourself with the same kindness and compassion that you offer to others. Learning to be kind to yourself during difficult times will allow you to find and affirm your intrinsic value.

The Importance of Kindness and Self-Compassion

Self-compassion is a simple skill that you can develop to ease your self-criticism and self-judgment. Learning to be kind and considerate to yourself as well as to others is crucial in the process of managing your stress and anxiety. Learning to quiet judgmental self-talk is very powerful, because when you no longer have to "listen" to this distracting negative commentary, you won't lose sight of your intrinsic value.

In the world of psychology, the idea of *kindness to yourself* is known as *self-compassion*, and it has received a lot of research attention. Self-compassion is the experience of extending kindness and caring toward yourself. It's a willingness to be moved by your own sorrow and pain; to take an understanding, nonjudgmental attitude toward your failures and shortfalls; and to see your experience as part of the overall human experience (Neff 2003).

Self-kindness, it turns out, is a powerful asset. Recent studies indicate that the ability to have self-compassion appears to reduce depression and anxiety (Neff, Kirkpatrick, and Rude 2007), and it may do so by reducing repetitive thinking and rumination (Raes 2010). Self-compassion also appears to motivate people to improve themselves (Breines and Chen 2012). It is associated with higher levels of happiness (Neff, Kirkpatrick, and Rude 2007) and may help explain why mindfulness is so effective. Self-compassion seems to be an important component of mindfulness's success for people with depression and anxiety (Van Dam et al. 2011). The next section will help you learn how to be kinder to yourself.

Working with Self-Compassion

Have you ever tried to say nice things to yourself when you are feeling anxious, only to discover that your words really don't work? That's because it takes more than nice words to address the problem. First, your body must relax and your worry thoughts need to slow. So the next time something makes you anxious, or you find yourself guided by fear, breathe long and deep for a minute. Then find a motivating, kind, and true statement of reassurance that can help shift the litany of self-doubt. Once you have calmed your breath, gently say to yourself, "I can be kind to myself. I can let self-compassion guide me." Next, acknowledge the facts of the situation at hand.

Here are some examples of self-compassion statements to say to yourself as you breathe deeply:

It's okay that I'm anxious. I can slow my breath and be kind to me.

It's okay that I am sad. Anyone would feel this way in this circumstance. It's part of the experience of being human.

Maybe I'm not reading the situation correctly. I can wait—I can suspend judgment. I can stay balanced and patient and wait to see what comes next.

Observing yourself with kindness and making use of statements such as these can move you toward a more self-compassionate inner reflection. You *can* honestly examine the areas where you need to grow and change without applying the false and limiting label of "failure" to yourself. Try shifting from "I always make mistakes" to "I have made a mistake, but I have the courage to try again." By enacting subtle shifts such as this, you will begin to build a greater sense of possibility for yourself, which can enhance both your self-confidence and your trust in your intrinsic value.

Use the following exercise to practice responding to your fears and self-doubts with kindness rather than criticism. Practicing this new habit here will help you begin to incorporate it into your daily life when things get hard.

EXERCISE:
Developing Self-Compassion

Sit up straight and tall in Easy Pose. Begin Long Deep Breathing (see Week 2).

1. Choose two self-compassion statements, such as ones from the previous page, and write them here:

   _____

   _____

2. Notice one of your milder self-criticisms and write it down as well:

   _____

3. Gently consider your self-compassion statements. Straighten your posture and breathe deeply. Notice how you feel and describe it below.

   _____

Throughout your day, try to become aware of the path your thoughts take when something challenging happens. Listen for those self-critical statements, and instead gently encourage yourself to say one of the self-compassion statements you wrote down. Take a long deep breath as you do this, to quiet and soothe the physical tension you are experiencing. Repeat to yourself that self-kindness is important to you—it's an *ideal by which you live your life*. Caring for yourself in this way and attending to your needs with self-compassion reminds you that you deserve to treat yourself well and that you have value.

The ability for self-compassion and for speaking and acting in accord with your intrinsic value requires a healthy nervous system. If our nervous system is not functioning well, neurotransmitters may not send proper signals to the brain, causing confusion and perhaps misinterpretation of events (Stahl 2008). Recognition of our intrinsic value and our ability to be compassionate with ourselves can be affected if our nervous system is not functioning well. An imbalanced nervous system sends signals to the glandular system that produces hormones related to depression and anxiety (Gard et al. 2014). The following yoga set is said to help improve glandular and nervous system activities. The first exercise is believed to stimulate the pituitary gland, which helps to create a balance between the parasympathetic and sympathetic nervous systems.

KY YOGA:
Set for Nervous System and Glandular Balance
(Bhajan 1983a, 35)

Sit in Easy Pose or in a chair with a straight back.

1. (A) Extend your arms straight out to the sides parallel to the ground, palms facing up.

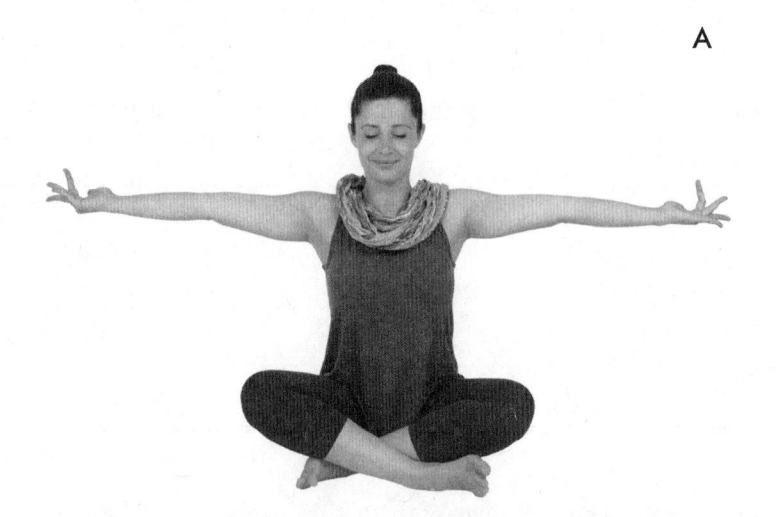

A

Begin to move only the middle finger up and down rapidly.

Using a powerful breath, inhale as you raise the finger and exhale as you lower it. Continue rhythmically, coordinating this movement with the breath.

Begin with 1 minute, and you can build to 7 minutes.

2. (B) Stretch your arms out in front, parallel to the ground, palms facing down.

Place your left hand over the right, interlacing the fingers.

Begin to swing your arms from side to side, moving the head and neck in the same direction as the arms, keeping the elbows straight.

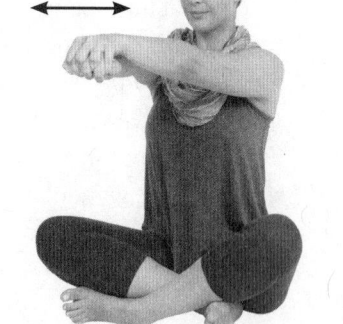

B

Continue coordinating the movement with a powerful breath.

Begin with 1 minute, and you can build to 5 minutes.

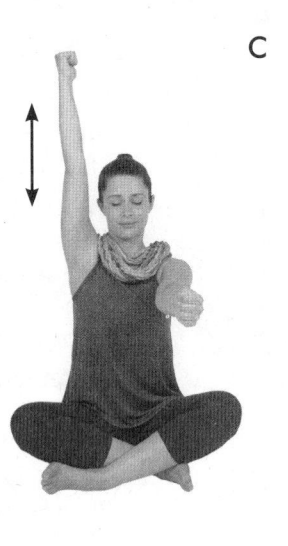

C

3. (C) Extend your arms straight out in front and parallel to the ground, palms facing each other.

    Make fists with your hands with the thumbs tucked inside, touching the fleshy mound below the little finger.

    Keeping the arms and hands straight, bring your left arm straight up over your head as the right arm goes down to reach a point parallel to the ground.

    Continue to alternate moving the arms up and down forcefully, coordinating the movement with forceful breathing.

    Begin with 1 minute, and you can build to 8 minutes.

4. (D) If you are sitting in a chair, please sit with your spine straight. If possible, bring the soles of your feet together.

    If sitting on the floor, sit with the soles of your feet pressed together, with your feet drawn into the groin.

D

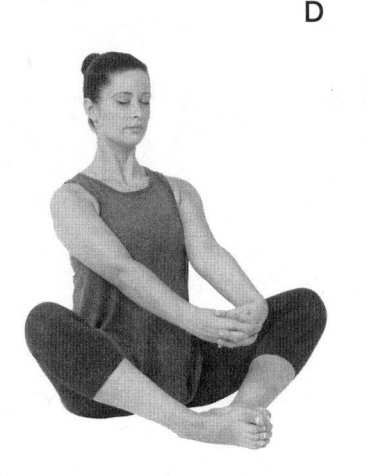

Keep your knees as close to the floor as possible.

Interlace your fingers and place your hands in your lap.

(E) Inhale and raise your arms over your head while simultaneously drawing the knees up toward the center of your body.

Exhale and lower the knees and arms down to the original position.

Continue this movement rhythmically, coordinating the movement with forceful breathing.

Begin with 1 minute, and you can build to 8 minutes.

Inhale and suspend the breath briefly. Exhale and relax the breath, relax the posture.

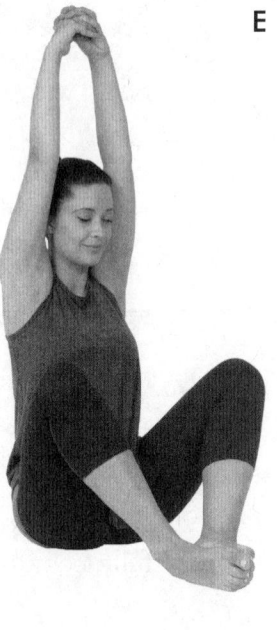

E

After you do this yoga set, relax for a minute or two and then begin Long Deep Breathing (see Week 2).

The concept of intrinsic value addresses your relationship with yourself and your personal sense of worth. The next concept, the *internal guidance system* (IGS), brings your attention to the principles that guide you in making choices based on concepts that are most important to you. Following these inspiring beliefs will lead you to a more fulfilled and happy life. When life gets hard, we are all stronger if we can hold on to our sense of personal value and to the important beliefs that guide us.

Your Internal Guidance System

An Internal Guidance System (IGS) is a set of principles from which we make decisions, take actions, and communicate. It directs mental habits and therefore has a huge impact on how we move through the world and view our lives. We all have an IGS, with rules that activate in different circumstances. It's helpful to become aware of the specific principles by which you are living currently and to consider whether there is a reason to shift the principles that guide your actions in your life.

When your IGS is healthy and strong, it will keep you moving along in a positive direction. Developing an approach that is based on the principles of wisdom, compassion, and competency is the goal for living a life that is happy and on course.

When your IGS is guided by automatic or unintended negative rules, a less successful route is taken. In the case of anxiety, fear often serves as the basis for your IGS. This often comes at a cost and leads to more anxiety, social isolation, and sadness as this type of IGS limits your decision-making process. For example, Marie, who struggles with anxiety, avoids returning to places where she has experienced anxious symptoms. One of them is the crowded shopping mall. Her IGS tells her to avoid anxiety-provoking situations because she can't cope with her symptoms. Fear is directing Marie's life and guiding her decisions and actions.

Use the exercise below to identify your negative IGS.

EXERCISE:
Identify Your Negative Internal Guidance System

Sit quietly and ask yourself these two questions. Write down your responses.

1. What negative beliefs guide me?

   _____

   _____

2. How do they affect my thoughts and actions?

   _____

   _____

Listen to how your thoughts reply when you ask these questions. If you do not hear a response, sit meditatively, do the One-Minute Breath (see Week 2), and again ask each question, slowly.

Once you have identified your negative IGS, you can learn to identify and shift to an IGS based in wisdom. Wise concepts can become guideposts for you as you begin to develop a more inspired and positive outlook. The following two meditations may help you incorporate these concepts more easily.

The first, Breath of Fire, is a special breathing exercise used in Kundalini Yoga. This breath is said to have many benefits including strengthening your nervous system, which prepares you to act more effectively, and increasing oxygen to the brain so that you can think in a more focused, clear, and neutral fashion (Bhajan 2003). It engages the navel point, which is located a few inches below the belly button in front of the lower spine.

KY MEDITATION:
Breath of Fire

(Bhajan 2003, 95)

When you practice Breath of Fire, the breath is guided by the relaxation and contraction of the navel point, which creates the rhythm for you to follow. The steady pace, along with the equally timed inhales and exhales, are important components of the breath. Once you learn Breath of Fire, it can be used with many other postures.

Sit in Easy Pose.

Place your hands in gyan mudra.

Focus on the point between the eyebrows.

Begin this meditation by panting through the mouth, like a puppy might.

Once the rhythm is established, close your mouth and continue to breathe in the same pattern but through your nose.

Continuously inhale and exhale without pausing (2 to 3 breaths per second). There is equal power given to the inhale and the exhale.

Begin with 1 minute, and build to 3 minutes.

To end: Inhale and hold for 10 seconds. Relax. Stay still for 1 minute, and you can build to 3 minutes. Watch the natural flow of the breath and the constant stream of internal and external sensations.

Inhale and suspend the breath briefly. Exhale and relax the breath, relax the posture.

The next meditation, Tune Up Your Thinking, uses Breath of Fire in a different way. It is said to specifically affect the frontal lobe of the brain (Bhajan and Khalsa 2006), which has many functions, including evaluating options and critical thinking. Kieran Fox and associates (2014) reviewed twenty-one neuroimaging studies involving a total of three hundred meditators and found that several areas of the brain were positively affected by meditation, including parts of the frontal lobe. Because the frontal lobe plays an important role in problem solving and decision making, the Tune Up Your Thinking meditation may help you evaluate your current guidance system and shift to a more uplifting one.

KY MEDITATION:
Tune Up Your Thinking

(Bhajan and Khalsa 2006, 80)

Sit in Easy Pose.

Close your eyes as you wish.

Extend your arms out in front at the shoulder level, parallel to the floor, with no bend in the elbows.

Your right palm faces up, and your left palm faces down.

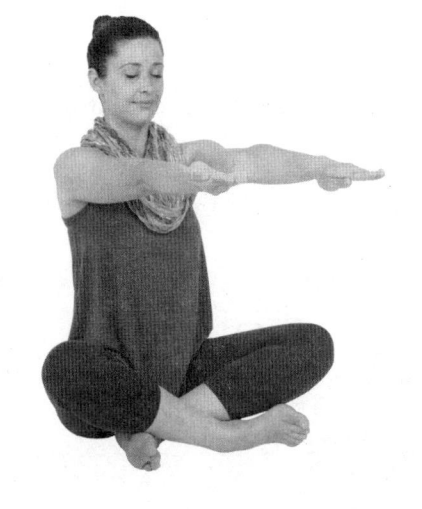

Hold the position and begin Breath of Fire (see previous meditation).

Start with 1 to 2 minutes, and you can build to 11 to 16 minutes.

To end: Hold the position; inhale and hold the breath for 15 seconds as you stretch the arms out in front and stretch your spine upward and tighten the muscles that hold the spine.

Pull the hands forward from the shoulders. Exhale.

Repeat this ending sequence of breathing and stretching two more times.

Inhale and suspend the breath briefly. Exhale and relax the breath, relax the posture.

Relax and do Long Deep Breathing for 2 minutes (see Week 2).

An Internal Guidance System Based in Wisdom

Wisdom is the ability to use one's experience, knowledge, insight, and good judgment in one's actions and decision making. Many writers throughout history have discussed the importance of wisdom as a touchstone in a life well led. Steven Covey, a popular and respected author in the fields of business and leadership, speaks of the importance of following a set of inspiring principles that can serve as a *moral compass* (Covey 1989; Covey 1992). He reminds us that the major world religions all teach that values such as honesty, integrity, patience, and charity should guide humanity. This is also true of yogic philosophy (Desikachar 1995). Yogi Bhajan, for example, often spoke of the importance of being a consistent, truthful, and trustworthy person who could live a principled life (Bhajan 2000).

Below is a list of universal and enduring qualities that exemplify wisdom and that represent humanity at its best:

Courage	Honesty	Service
Peace	Patience	Dignity
Kindness	Grace	Sincerity

Do you recognize aspects of yourself in this list? You probably already possess some of these qualities, though you may not realize it. Or you might aspire toward some of them. You can use the following exercise to identify the wisdom-based concepts that are important to you.

EXERCISE:
Identify Your Wisdom-Based Internal Guidance System

Sit quietly and reflect on the list of enduring qualities. Then answer the following questions.

1. Which wisdom-based qualities do I possess?

    _____

    _____

    _____

2. How have I experienced one or more of these qualities in my life?

    _____

    _____

    _____

3. How do these qualities affect my thoughts and actions?

    _____

    _____

    _____

4. Are there new qualities that I would like to incorporate in my IGS?

    _____

    _____

    _____

5. How would these new qualities affect my thoughts and actions?

    _____

    _____

    _____

Now that you have completed this task, the next step is to adopt these wise concepts as *principles* to guide your choices. Once you make this shift and begin to live in alignment with the principles that you value, you will find that you feel better about yourself.

Principles as Habits

Once you begin to accept that *you can take control* of what guides you, you're better able to approach the challenges in your life proactively. You can respond to life from the strength of your principles rather than defensively reacting to stress from a position of fear.

For example, when faced with a stressful situation, you can learn to *choose courage* as your guide in that moment, rather than allowing the automatic fear response to take control. This doesn't mean that you aren't afraid; it simply means that you choose to be directed by courage rather than fear. With attention and practice, your guiding principles will become habits.

When this transformation occurs, ideals such as courage and kindness become more important than fear or sadness. Choose to place these and similar principles at the center of your IGS, and make wisdom the touchstone for the habits you create.

Over time, when you repeatedly choose wisdom over a negative, reactive emotion, you are more likely to *like* the person you are and how you behave. This authenticity will create a kind of radiance, and you'll see other people respond to it in positive ways.

As you can imagine, if you could always align yourself with these principles, you'd become the person you want to be—calm, strong, kind, and honest. Each success will serve to reinforce the new self-concept. When principle-guided decision making becomes a habit, you create a new internal structure from which to interact with the world. You will create a calm place, with a bedrock guidance system filled with integrity and strength.

The following exercise uses breath and posture along with self-reflection to help you create new mental habits and shift your IGS to one that is based on wisdom.

EXERCISE:
Shifting Your Internal Guidance System

It's important to gently acknowledge old habits and fears before you focus on creating new habits. It's easier to make a change when you shift both your body and your mind. Noticing your breath and your posture will physically support the mental changes you are making. Write your responses in the space provided.

1. Identify an anxious mental habit you would like to change:

   _____

2. Identify what is guiding this habit. Is it fear or something else?

   _____

3. Notice the breathing pattern associated with this habit.

4. Sit up straight and correct your breath using Long Deep Breathing (see Week 2) for 1 minute.

5. Focus on the wise principle you chose earlier and write it here:

   _____

6. Notice your breath, and maintain a natural breath.

7. Ask yourself how you will act differently based on your chosen principle. Write it here:

   _____

8. Now pay attention to how you feel.

Were you able to notice and shift an anxious habit? If not, don't feel discouraged—if you keep practicing, you will see changes in your mental habits over time.

It is within your power to make shifts toward a more positive and self-supporting internal dialogue. Learn to listen to the things that you repeat to yourself and to what guides your thoughts and actions. Remember that the way your body feels when you are struggling will affect the way you think. Notice your breath, and gently remind yourself to breathe long and deep when you are stressed and your body needs to relax. Over time, acknowledging your intrinsic value and allowing your wisdom-based IGS to guide you will bring you greater self-acceptance and joy.

The next meditation is said to affect the pituitary gland, which controls the function of several other endocrine glands (Chapman 2016). When these glands are not functioning properly, we feel tired, irritable, and less able to act in ways that are consistent with our goals. The pituitary gland also affects our ability to evaluate outcomes and choose between different options (Collins and Koechlin 2012). Therefore, an improved pituitary function makes it is easier for us to choose actions that are consistent with our valued principles and our desired character.

KY MEDITATION:
To Control Your Character
(Bhajan and Khalsa 2006, 127)

Sit in Easy Pose.

Press the thumb on each of your hands against the mound at the base of the pinkie finger.

Close your fingers around the thumb, making a tight fist. Your thumbs should feel very pressurized.

Press your fists together so the second segments of the backs of your fingers on each hand are touching the corresponding second segments of the other hand. The backs of your thumbs are facing your chest.

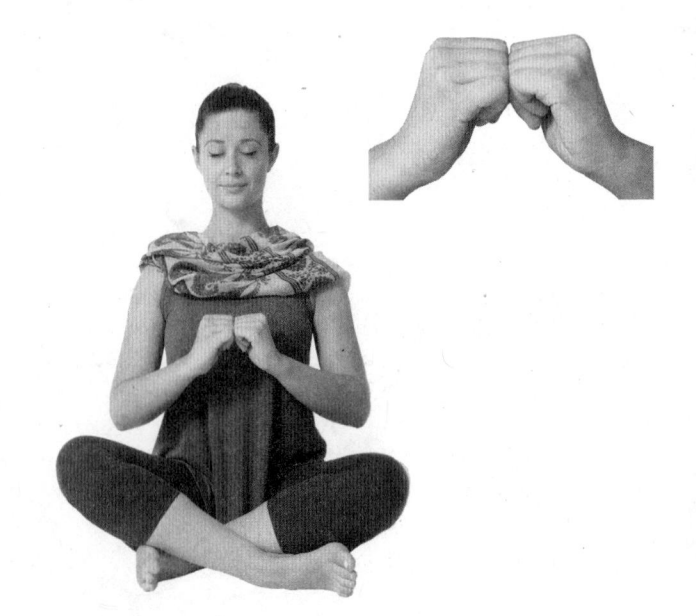

Bend your elbows so they rest at your sides and so that your hands are level with the heart center and a few inches from your body.

Let your eyes look at the tip of your nose.

Inhale through your nose (4 seconds).

Exhale through your mouth (4 seconds).

Inhale through your mouth (4 seconds).

Exhale through your nose (4 seconds).

Continue consciously and rhythmically alternating the breath between your nose and your mouth in this way.

Begin with 1 to 3 minutes, and build to 11 minutes.

To end: Inhale deeply to your maximum. Hold 15 to 20 seconds as you really stretch your spine, arms, and hands upward. Stretch as if you are trying to lift yourself off the ground. Exhale and repeat the ending sequence of the breathing and stretching motion two more times.

Inhale and suspend the breath briefly. Exhale and relax the breath, relax the posture.

After finishing this meditation, sit quietly for a minute or two, breathing long and deep. Focus on the point between your eyebrows and listen to the sound of your breath and then relax.

Throughout this book, you have been working to progressively develop skills to manage anxiety in your mind and body, and to enhance your self-view. The final section of this chapter will help you bring all of these concepts together to create a new framework for your positive self-view.

Working with Cognitive Distortions and Negative Self-View

As we have discussed in this chapter, when we are anxious, our thoughts can run in negative and self-critical directions that can lead us to distort the facts of a situation. Left unchallenged, this thought pattern makes us feel anxious and depressed. Collectively, these inaccurate ways of thinking are referred to in CBT as *cognitive distortions* (Beck 1995).

Cognitive distortions often become more frequent and more pronounced during periods of stress and anxiety, negatively coloring one's self-view. The following table captures the ten most common types of cognitive distortion.

Cognitive Distortions (Beck 1995)

All or nothing	You think in absolutes, black or white.
Overgeneralization	You view one negative event as a never-ending pattern of defeat: "This *always* happens."
Mental filter	You dwell on the negatives and ignore the positives.
Discounting the positive	You insist that your positive qualities don't count.
Jumping to conclusions	You jump to conclusions not warranted by the facts:
• Mind reading	• You assume that people are reacting negatively to you.
• Fortune-telling	• You predict things will turn out badly.
Magnification and minimization	You blow things out of proportion or shrink them.
Emotional reasoning	You reason from your emotions: "I *feel* like an idiot, so I must really *be* one."
Should statements	You use the words "should," "shouldn't," "must," "ought," and "have to."
Labeling	Instead of saying, "I made a mistake," you say, "I'm a jerk" or "I'm a loser."
Blame	You find fault instead of solving the problem:
• Self-blame	• You blame yourself for something you weren't entirely responsible for.
• Other blame	• You blame others and overlook ways you contributed to the problem.

On the following pages you will find a worksheet that will, first, help you identify the self-beliefs that are central to your negative self-view. It will also prompt you to actively identify which cognitive distortions support your negative self-view and subsequent anxiety.

Y-CBT WORKSHEET:
Who Am I?

Self-Belief: In the left column, list the self-beliefs that are most problematic for you. Consider the beliefs that negatively affect your view of yourself, and perhaps your relationships, because of your struggles with anxiety.

Distortions: In the center column, identify the cognitive distortions that help you to question the negative self-beliefs that you have listed (refer to the Cognitive Distortions table on the preceding page).

Y-CBT Alternatives: In the right column, list the Y-CBT techniques or practices that you can use to respond to your concern in a self-supportive and compassionate way. After you complete the worksheet, you will uncover a more compassionate self-view.

Who Am I? Write down your name, then identify a word or quality that you would like to associate with yourself that illustrates your finest attribute. This may be one of your intrinsic values or a principle that guides your wisdom-based IGS.

An Image: As a final step in this process, choose an image that captures the fine quality that you have selected to associate with your name. Having this visual symbol anchors and solidifies the concept that you are capturing for yourself. It could be something from nature, an animal, or simply a color. You can draw it or find an image in a magazine or on the web.

EXAMPLE Y-CBT WORKSHEET
Who Am I?

Self-Belief	Distortions	Y-CBT Alternatives
1. I'm not good enough. 2. I fail at most things I try.	All or nothing Overgeneralization Jumping to conclusions Magnification and minimization Emotional reasoning Labeling	1. I can remind myself of my strengths and my intrinsic values of intelligence and hard work to remember that I can be victorious, even though I sometimes make mistakes. 2. I can talk to myself with kindness, and I can sit with a straight spine, in a posture of love and victory. 3. I can sit up straight, take a few deep breaths, be in the moment, and remember: "I'll be okay. Everything will be all right."

Who am I?

_Sarah_____   _Resilient_____
           (my name)   (quality)

. An image that represents my quality:

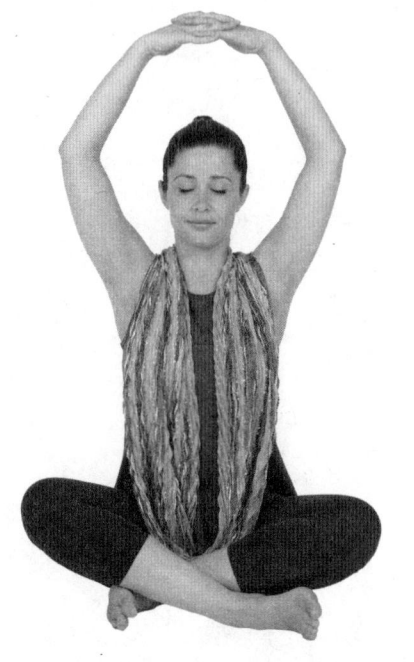

Y-CBT WORKSHEET:
Who Am I?

Self-Belief	Distortions	Y-CBT Alternatives

Who am I?

_____   _____
          (my name)   (quality)

An image that represents my quality:

In Summary

We hope that this chapter has helped to make you more aware of your intrinsic value. You have explored the positive, unchanging qualities that are present in you, regardless of the struggles that you may face. You have also considered your internal compass and the inspiring principles that can guide your decision making. Following these positive principles and this new awareness will bring you to a place of self-pride and self-worth. Challenging the negative beliefs you have held on to and replacing them with a sense of hope and possibility will help free you from anxiety and move you toward a quieter and more peaceful attitude.

Week 4 Daily Y-CBT Practice

Guiding Principle

Habits of mind influence our lives. What we think affects how we feel. Our thoughts are of our own making. Because we are the only ones who are thinking our thoughts, we can choose to create habits of the mind that give us peace and victory.

Yoga and Meditation

1. Set for Nervous System and Glandular Balance

2. Tune Up Your Thinking

3. To Control Your Character

Daily Living Practice

Your practice this week is to focus on your intrinsic value and become clear about your personal sense of innate worth, which is unchanging regardless of the challenges you face in life. We also invite you to become aware of and strengthen a set of core inspirational principles, or your IGS, that guides you in your life choices. To internalize these concepts, complete and practice the following exercises:

- Identify your intrinsic value: Begin your list with three positive attributes. Add to the list each day, after you do your yoga and meditation practice.

- Identify your wisdom-based internal guidance system.

- Complete the Y-CBT Worksheet: Who Am I? using Y-CBT alternatives.

Daily Practice Log

	Sunday		Monday		Tuesday		Wednesday		Thursday		Friday		Saturday	
Time of Day														
	B	A	B	A	B	A	B	A	B	A	B	A	B	A
Yoga/Meditation I Used														
Y-CBT Techniques I Used														

B = Before, A = After

1	2	3	4	5	6	7	8	9	10

Low Anxiety   Moderate Anxiety   High Anxiety

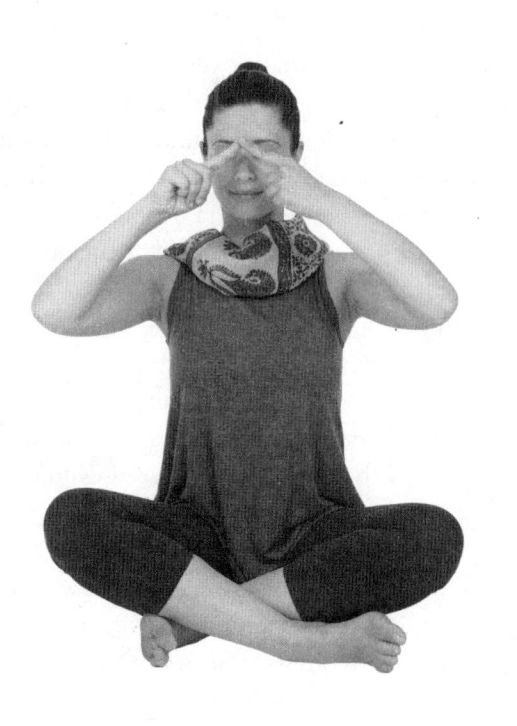

WEEK 5

Strengthening Communication:
The Reciprocal Loop

Communication is a *reciprocal loop*, a back-and-forth interaction, between individuals. Communication creates a shared experience through a mutual interchange of thought and feeling. When communication is flowing well, it's like a graceful dance; participants move in rhythm with each other, and the coordination and connection create good feelings. When communication is not going well, it's still a dance of action and reaction, just not a pleasant one; people are out of sync, stepping on each other's toes and bumping into each other. For better or for worse, communication has a huge impact on both the speaker and the listener.

Throughout this chapter, we invite you to consider the following Y-CBT guiding principle: **There is a "reciprocal loop" in all communication.** In every encounter between individuals, there is a back-and-forth interaction that creates the mood and the message between the participants. Awareness and ownership of how we influence our interactions is profoundly important in the development of healthy and satisfying relationships. This means that the simple act of attending to ourselves—our body, our breath, our thoughts—with nurturing acceptance and encouragement is a powerful mechanism for change. It is also important that we understand the underlying goals of our thoughts, words, and actions.

Communication is a full mind-body experience. People interpret what you say not only through your words but also through the nonverbal, sensory cues that accompany those words, including your facial expressions, rhythm of speech, gestures, breathing patterns, posture, tone of voice, and eye contact. We routinely read these small sensory cues and respond to them. At the same time, we are also giving off nonverbal cues, which the other person is interpreting and responding to. Our brains and biochemistry are hard at work interpreting both our own feelings and experience and also what might be going on in the other person.

In this chapter, we share some ideas to help you examine how anxiety affects your communication style, and you will work on acquiring some new skills to reduce the impact of anxiety while improving the way you communicate with others. Some of these skills are *intrapersonal* in nature, that is, within yourself. They include awareness of your intentions, acting according to your values, and having an authentic, compassionate presence. Other skills are more *interpersonal* in nature, that is, related to what happens between you and others. They include understanding how you present to others, your ability to interpret their emotions, and your ability to create feelings of connection and understanding.

Y-CBT is a progressive journey of self-growth. In previous chapters, we talked about ways to work on your internal dialogue. Now we'll apply the same principles to the complex world of human interaction. Using your new knowledge, you will be able to develop skills for building happier, healthier, and more authentic relationships.

We'll begin with an exploration of the surprising biochemical-emotional processes that underlie social understanding.

Biochemistry and Social Awareness

Throughout the twentieth century, theorists wrote about social awareness, and the concept was popularized by Daniel Goleman in the 1990s with his best-selling book *Emotional Intelligence: Why It Can Matter More Than IQ* (1995). During the past few decades, many theories about social awareness have been developed, and the concept has received significant research attention under various designations, such as social intelligence, emotional intelligence, social cognition, social neuropsychology, and cognitive neuropsychology.

One of the interesting ideas common to these theoretical models is that physical cues (also called social cues) actually trigger biochemical and neurological reactions not only in the person speaking but in the listener as well. On some level, awareness of these sensory cues coordinates with neurological chemistry to create our lived experience of our social world (Critchley 2009; Goleman 2004; Kassin, Fein, and Markus 2008).

This research has shaped the way we think about communication today because we understand that there is more than just words at play when we communicate: our body language, patterns of speech, and the way we connect with each other are based more on our physical and neurological patterns than we ever imagined.

By becoming more aware of these connections within yourself, you can heighten your ability to deal with the anxiety you feel when you communicate with others. The exercise below will help you deepen this awareness as you focus on the thoughts, fears, and physical sensations you experience in social settings.

EXERCISE:
Awareness of My Response to My Social World

Sit in Easy Pose and begin Long Deep Breathing (see Week 2) for 2 minutes. Then write down your answers to the following questions.

What is happening in my social world right now? Am I happy with it? If not, how would I want it to be different?

_____

_____

_____

_____

What is happening to me physically as I think about my social life?

_____

_____

How would I want my body to feel? _____

_____

_____

Is anxiety impacting my interactions, my social life, or my work life?

_____

_____

_____

Shifting your outlook will help you begin to engage more authentically with others and reduce some of your automatic fear of interacting with other people, which, left unchecked, can develop into serious social anxiety.

Working with Social Anxiety

Social settings can arouse anxiety in any of us from time to time. This discomfort can arise for many reasons. Some people have a pervasive fear that others won't like them or that they won't fit in. Others feel unprepared for an unknown situation and react anxiously to that unfamiliarity. Still others can't shake the fear that they might do something to embarrass themselves in front of other people.

Social anxiety, or the experience of fear in the presence of other people, is one of the most common forms of anxiety. In the United States, up to 7 percent of the population has this experience (American Psychiatric Association 2013). It may be helpful to focus on the fact that you aren't "the only person at the party" who is anxious! Sometimes, just reminding yourself of this point can open a pathway to relief.

Social anxiety can cause feelings of dread, fear of humiliation, or racing thoughts fueled by negative self-beliefs or doubts. Physical symptoms might include shaking, sweating, light-headedness, stuttering, or confusion (American Psychiatric Association 2013).

If you struggle in social settings, it's likely that a couple of things are going on. First, cognitive distortions (discussed in the previous chapter) may emerge, causing you to negatively "predict" the outcome of your next social experience. Remember the concept of anticipatory anxiety from Week 2? Such predictions are a prime example of that. You might be telling yourself that the next experience will be the same as an unpleasant one you had in the past: "I always choke up when I talk to new people," or "People always think I am weird because I have an accent." Or perhaps, based on your negative beliefs about yourself, you enter the setting by automatically putting yourself in a "one-down" position, comparing yourself unfavorably to others: "Everyone else in the room is smarter, prettier, funnier, or richer than me."

Second, remember that the fear response, if left unchecked, will cause you to momentarily hold your breath or over-breathe. You will retain carbon dioxide, which will cause physical symptoms such as tremulousness, light-headedness, a racing heart, and confusion.

In the previous exercise, you practiced becoming aware of your responses in social situations. This awareness is key to breaking the reactive pattern that has become a habit for you. Your challenge now is to move away from reactivity and toward a mindful, intentional approach to the situation. You can learn to quiet your automatic negative reactions and replace them with a quiet, proactive, and self-supporting response.

Anxiety causes people to leave the present moment and begin to have worried thoughts, such as "What should I say next? What is the other person thinking? How do I look to the other person?" The next time this happens to you, try turning your mind from those thoughts and bringing yourself into a state of relaxation by asking yourself these questions instead: "Is my breathing slow and peaceful? Is my posture comfortable but straight? Can I be gentle with myself and the other person?" It's surprising but true: when you are anxious while communicating with others, relaxation is the remedy.

Professional athletes are often encouraged to visualize and mentally rehearse how they hope to perform in competition (Newmark 2012). For example, a baseball batter might be advised to mentally rehearse hitting a home run. This visualization is said to activate physiological processes that are similar to those that would occur if the player was on the playing field.

In the next exercise, we invite you to mentally practice feeling relaxed in a social situation. The next time you are fearful about meeting a friend, try this technique. Then, when you are with the friend, check in on your breath to see how you are doing. If your breathing is not relaxed, change it and use self-compassion statements such as those found in Week 4. You can measure your success by how often you are able to remain relaxed.

EXERCISE:
Mental Rehearsal to Reduce Anxiety

This exercise will help you avert anxious feelings if you practice it before you meet with someone who might make you uncomfortable.

1. Think of a person you might see in the near future who might cause you to feel anxious.

2. Visualize how the person will look, and picture a typical setting where you might see him or her. Next, simply notice how you feel.

3. How is your breathing?

    _____

4. What is your posture?

    _____

5. What are you thinking?

    _____

    _____

6. Begin to calm your body. Slow your breath and feel yourself breathe through your whole body—from your toes to your head. Straighten your posture. Sit up comfortably with a straight spine, with your shoulders lined up over your hips.

7. Picture yourself in a comfortable, relaxed, and confident state in the presence of this person. Breathe and note how this feels in your body.

8. Keep in mind that the more relaxed you feel, the better your chances for a good interaction. You can remind yourself that relaxation is a cure. You can use wisdom and self-compassion to gently encourage yourself. You can remember your intrinsic value.

Using mental rehearsal to prepare yourself for stressful social situations can help you to reduce your anxiety and thereby communicate in more relaxed and successful ways.

The next yoga set is designed to help you develop more accurate intuition and the confidence to speak your own truth. Many anxious people report that it helps them speak from their heart. You will see that the set begins with an exercise that puts your whole body in motion. Through these movements, you will physically and mentally begin to loosen up. Then you stretch out your arms, opening the heart center, which, in yogic theory, gives you more compassion. Allow your breath to adjust itself for the first two parts, and follow the instructions for the breath in the final segment and to finish. Working the breath is said to improve the functioning of the parasympathetic nervous system, which helps calm and relax you (Streeter et al. 2012).

KY YOGA:
Set for Heart, Voice, and Intuition
(Bhajan 1997)

1. Sit in Easy Pose or in a chair with your spine straight and tall.

    Open your eyes and look straight ahead.

    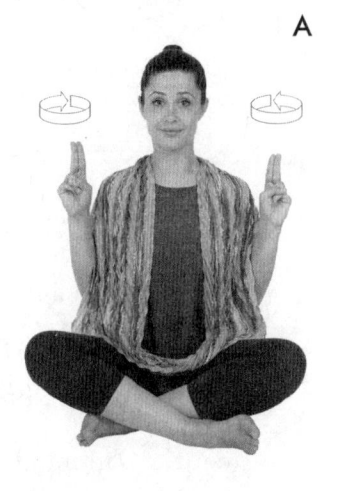

    (A) Using your thumb, lock down the pinkie and the finger next to it on each hand.

    Your other fingers point straight up.

    Bend your elbows and press them tightly into the sides of your rib cage. This will allow your whole body to move as the hands revolve.

    Revolve your hands rapidly in small circles, 3 cycles per second. Keep moving them without stopping.

    Begin with 1 minute, and you can build to 5.5 minutes.

    To remember: If you are doing this correctly, your spine and shoulders will loosen up too. It is also good for your heart and your brain.

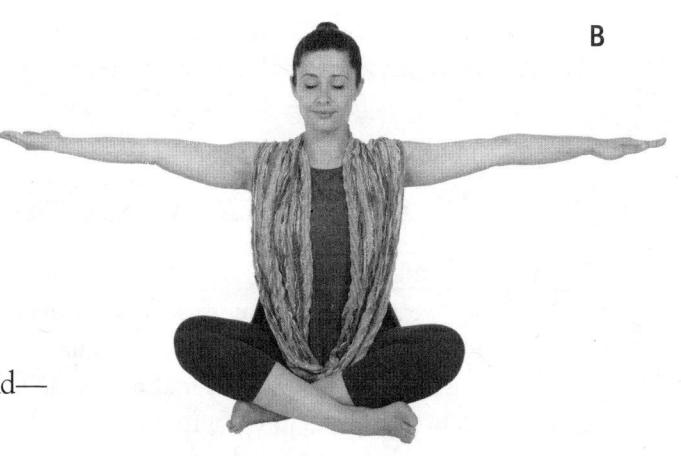

2. (B) Stretch your arms out to the sides, without bending your elbows. Your right palm faces up, left palm faces down.

    Close your eyes and focus on the tip of your nose.

    Let your body balance itself.

    Become very still and try to be solid—like a stone. Sit without moving.

    Begin with 1 minute, and you can build to 6 minutes.

3. (C) Inhale and clasp your hands together, interlacing your fingers.

    Lift your arms up to form a circle over the top of your head.

    Keep your eyes closed.

    Exhale. Hold this position and whistle an enjoyable tune.

    Begin with 1 minute, and you can build to 6 minutes.

    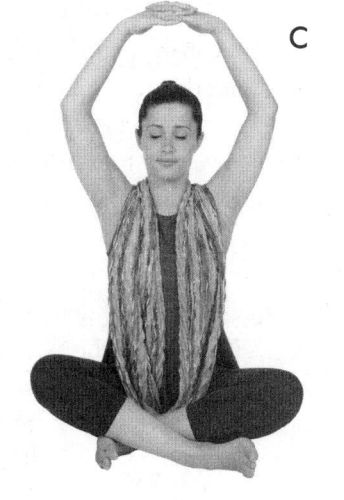

    To end: Inhale and hold your breath for 15 seconds while stretching your arms higher, lifting up your entire body, and expanding the rib cage outward.

    Then exhale.

    Inhale, hold the breath for 10 seconds, and stretch upward. Open the chest cavity as wide as possible.

    Exhale.

    For the last time: Inhale and hold your breath for 10 seconds while slowly and strongly twisting to the left and then to the right.

    Return to center, exhale, and relax.

    Inhale and suspend the breath briefly. Exhale and relax the breath, relax the posture.

    When you finish, practice Long Deep Breathing (see Week 2) for 1 to 2 minutes.

Remember, change takes time. Be patient, keep practicing, and be kind to yourself. In time, you will find you are more attuned to yourself and to others.

How Anxiety Affects Communication

When anxiety affects our thoughts and feelings it has a direct impact on how we interact with other people. When we are anxious, our experience of distress causes us to focus inward, on ourselves, rather than outward, on what is actually going on around us. Anxious thoughts cause us to create stories and scenarios that may not be accurate and may include distortions. We believe the things we repeat to ourselves again and again, and eventually we may come to believe that our imaginings of what some-one else *might* be thinking or feeling about us are true.

In communication, this tendency can evolve into an automatic process of reacting to the thoughts we are having, rather than responding in a genuine, interactive way to the actual situation. When we communicate based on these anxious "theories," it becomes nearly impossible to have an authentic exchange with another person.

There are many ways anxiety can distort communication. When an anxious person enters a room, his or her physical presentation, eye contact, and tone of speaking are affected by how he or she is feeling, which in turn influences the interaction.

Consider Mary, a recent college graduate who found her first job in a small business. She is smart and capable, and was hired because of her abilities. Mary, however, has a long history of anxiety. She regularly questions even her proven abilities and critically compares her work to that of others. Mary has come to believe that she is always "less than" other people, and so she worries that other people believe this too. In her interactions with others at work, she *unconsciously* seeks confirmation of her negative theories about herself.

Because Mary erroneously believes she is inferior, she behaves in a way that conveys this. Even though she is smart and capable, she presents as tenuous and overly apologetic for minor errors. She questions every decision she makes. Her anxious comportment causes her coworkers to respond to her as if she lacks the skills to do the job. When she is passed over for new projects, Mary says to herself, "See, it's true; I am not as good as other people." This cycle then fuels further worry and confirms her negative self-beliefs. She withdraws from her coworkers, and her work performance suffers further, which increases her anxiety. And so the cycle continues.

Mary's situation illustrates one way that anxiety affects behavior and communication. In other instances, individuals who struggle with social anxiety have a difficult time making eye contact; speak in short, clipped sentences; and end conversations as quickly as possible. People may perceive this behavior as rudeness.

Still others experiencing great discomfort might unknowingly present as loud, demanding, and aggressive in an attempt to get through a situation, and then feel attacked and misunderstood when others respond to them in a defensive and hostile way.

People who struggle with anxiety are typically baffled, confused, and hurt by the responses they receive in these situations. They're so consumed by how they feel that they're blind to the way they are behaving and being perceived by others. This creates the experience of feeling chronically misunderstood, and, as in Mary's situation, the anxious person interprets this as confirmation of her own negative beliefs about herself.

Because of these factors, those who struggle with anxiety often experience themselves as "recipients" or even victims of their communications with others. Without having a clear understanding of what you're bringing to the interaction, you will *regularly feel out of control* in these situations. Learning your role in your communications will empower you to take new steps toward managing your anxious feelings and behaviors, which, as you may recall, is the premise of the guiding principle for this week. This self-understanding will help you work toward developing a more authentic and genuine communication style.

The following exercises are designed to help you take a close look at yourself in social situations. Consider each question with self-compassion and with the goal of gaining a greater understanding of what you bring to your interactions with others. You can't change without knowing what needs to be changed. Becoming aware of how you feel, behave, and present to others when you're anxious will set the stage for positive change.

If you find that you start to criticize yourself during the exercises, take a few moments to practice Long Deep Breathing (see Week 2) or Powering Down to Transform Anxiety (see Week 3) to create a more neutral state of mind.

EXERCISE:
What Does the "Anxious You" Look Like?

Take a moment and ask yourself the following questions:

What do my face and body express when I am anxious?

Do I smile? Frown or grimace?

Does my facial expression match how I feel?

How is my posture?

Is my speech rapid or halting?

Is my tone of voice very loud? Very soft?

Am I tenuous? Demanding?

Do I try to make myself "invisible"?

Do I talk too much so that no one asks me a question?

Do I make eye contact?

Write an honest description of how you think you appear and how you communicate when you are feeling stressed or anxious:

_____

_____

_____

Consider for a moment that you are in a conversation with the "anxious you." Describe how it might feel to be in a conversation with that person:

_____

_____

_____

Remember that statements containing the words *always* and *never* are rarely accurate. You are not *always* anxious, and it isn't true that you *never* feel comfortable in social situations. Anxiety and its partner self-criticism will cause you to draw these overarching negative conclusions about yourself, and if you repeat them enough, you will begin to believe they are true. The actual truth is probably that *sometimes* you are anxious and *sometimes* you are not.

Now that you understand how anxiety affects your communication style, you will begin to notice when these responses are happening. Then you can shift your breathing, redirect your thinking to facts, or even take a few minutes to meditate.

The following exercise asks you to attend to how you look, feel, and behave when you *aren't anxious*. It's important to remember that you aren't always anxious. You already possess many of the strengths you need to move through the times when you are feeling anxious. So pay close attention to the times when you are feeling strong and confident. You can learn to bring these strengths to difficult situations when you need them most!

EXERCISE:
What Does the "Calm You" Look Like?

Write down an example of a time when you were *not* anxious and you spoke in a calm way:

_____

_____

What were you feeling before you began to talk?

My emotions were: _____

_____.

My posture was: _____

_____.

My breath was: _____.

My intention was: _____.

Why do you think you were not anxious in this situation?

_____

_____

You are developing an awareness of the differences in your physical and emotional states when you are anxious and when you feel comfortable and confident. Hold on to this awareness. Become cognizant of the situations that cause you greater levels of anxiety, and use your new strategies to shift your response. Remember, you are in charge of your view of yourself. Holding on to your intrinsic value in social settings will help you interact with others in a more genuine and confident way.

Intrinsic Value and Communication

Sometimes we find ourselves in relationships that are painful or problematic. Often in these relationships, a *negative* reciprocal loop develops: exchanges with the other person generate an unpleasant feedback cycle that reinforces our insecurities and fears. In these situations, we often doubt our own value and judge ourselves based on the negative or even abusive behavior of others. Thus, it is critical that you learn to hold on to your sense of intrinsic value, as you identified in Week 4. And then, regardless of how others behave, you will be able to move through difficult interactions with your positive self-regard intact.

Difficult family or romantic relationships and stressful workplace relationships sometimes cause us to question our own view of ourselves, because those relationships (and those people) are profoundly important to us. When you find someone voicing a negative assessment of you, try to remember that it is simply *his* or *her* opinion—and just because someone says it doesn't make it so. Don't let it override your own self-view. Instead, ask yourself, "Do I agree? What is my opinion of myself here?"

If you base your opinion of yourself and your value solely on the behavior and words of others, you leave yourself emotionally vulnerable. This is a common and inherent trap in many relationships. But remember, your value exists *intrinsically*, regardless of the criticism of others. It is your responsibility to define and hold on to your value in the world during these moments.

This does not mean that it isn't important to take in the feedback of others and use it to support your personal growth, but if you place your *value as a person* in the pocket of another person, your experience of your own value is vulnerable.

Keep your value in your *own* pocket. Own it and regularly assess it. Know what your strengths and challenges are. Apply your own opinion of yourself in difficult interactions.

The following exercise will help you practice this important habit.

EXERCISE:
Keep Your Value "in Your Pocket"

You can reduce your emotional vulnerability in challenging relationships if you practice holding on to your view of yourself. This exercise can help you learn to keep your value in your own pocket rather then handing it over to another person.

Consider a situation when you were criticized by another person and describe it here:

_____

_____

What was the other person's opinion that challenged your belief in your intrinsic value?

_____

_____

What was your opinion that supported your belief in your intrinsic value?

_____

_____

Compare the two. What is your truth about yourself?

_____

_____

Is there anything useful that you can take away from the other person's opinion?

_____

_____

List the intrinsic values that support your self-view:

_____

_____

We hope these exercises have helped you see that your opinion of yourself is just as important, if not more so, than the opinion of a harsh or critical companion. Be your own advocate. Hold on to what you know to be true about yourself.

The emotional pain and anger that can arise from a difficult relationship can be hard to shake and can fuel your anxiety. If you struggle with such feelings, the following two meditations may help.

The first is the meditation Burn Inner Anger. This breathing exercise is done with a powerful breath. It can help you release some of the anger that prevents you from working through relationship conflicts.

The second meditation, Heal a Broken Heart, is designed to relax the autonomic nervous system and calm the breath, heart, and mind. The hand position is intended to create physical and energetic balance. In yogic theory this meditation is associated with healing a broken heart because "to heal the emotional wounds of the heart, we need to bring calm to the nerves that hold the wound. We know that a break in relationship (to others or to our self) has almost identical reactions in the nervous system and brain as a physical injury or loss of limb" (Bhajan 2009, 82).

KY MEDITATION:
Burn Inner Anger

(Bhajan and Khalsa 2006, 147)

Sit in Easy Pose with your spine straight. Chin in, chest out.

Close your eyes.

Extend your middle and index fingers of your right hand up, and use your thumb to hold down the other fingers.

Raise your right arm in front and up to 60 degrees. Your elbow is straight.

Place your left hand at your heart center.

Make an "O" of your mouth and inhale and exhale through your mouth (2-second inhalation, 2-second exhalation).

Breathe powerfully and with emotion. Burn your inner anger.

Begin with 1 minute, and you can build to 11 minutes.

To end: Inhale deeply and hold for 10 seconds. Stretch both arms up over your head and stretch your spine as much as you can. Stretch the discs between the vertebrae. Exhale like cannon fire. Repeat this ending breathing and stretching sequence twice more.

Inhale and suspend the breath briefly. Exhale and relax the breath, relax the posture.

Move smoothly into the next meditation.

KY MEDITATION:
Heal a Broken Heart
(Bhajan 2009, 82)

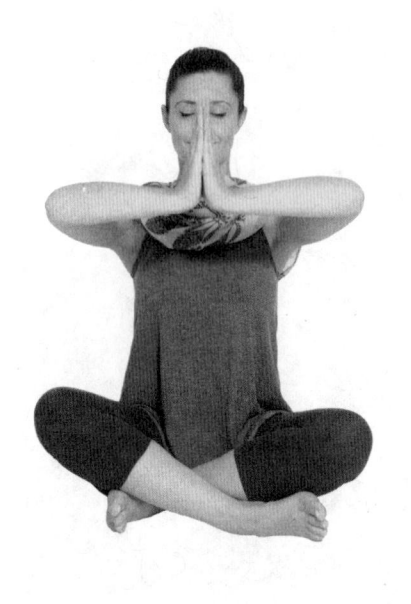

Sit in Easy Pose with a straight spine and neck. Look within.

Put your palms together, lightly touching.

Hold the tip of the middle fingers level with the point between your eyebrows. Your forearms are horizontal to the ground, and your elbows are high.

Allow your autonomic system to relax and your breath will automatically move toward a meditative pace to renew and relax your heart and mind.

Begin with 1 to 3 minutes, and you can build to 11, 31, or 62 minutes.

To end: Inhale, exhale, relax the breath, and with clasped hands stretch the arms up for 2 minutes.

Inhale and suspend the breath briefly. Exhale and relax the breath, relax the posture.

Using these meditations when you are struggling with emotional pain or anger can help calm your mind and body, and release some of those troubling emotions. The resulting quiet state will allow you greater clarity in working through the issues in the relationship. Each action you choose to make in interacting with the other person will affect his or her reaction. You can alter the relational dynamic by changing your behavior and emotional posture. This concept is called the reciprocal loop.

The Reciprocal Loop

In every human interaction there is a feedback loop. The words and actions of one person will always affect the words and actions of another person. Learning to understand and take full ownership of what you bring to each interaction you have is critical to the development of healthy and satisfying relationships.

Each interaction involves many elements that go beyond words. Each person has a *presence* in the exchange. As we noted earlier, this involves many physical factors and movements, along with the words that we speak. We are never simply "spoken to" in communication. Regardless of who is doing the talking at any given moment, there is an exchange that includes the responsiveness of the listener, which influences what is happening between both people and impacts the next word and action of the other. Each person responds and reacts, and the dialogue evolves as two people interact with one another. This back-and-forth exchange is what we call the *reciprocal loop*.

The next exercise is designed to give you an example of the warm reciprocity of human connection in its simplest form.

EXERCISE:
Pure, Positive Human Connection

Close your eyes and visualize an infant child whom you have known, and then picture yourself smiling at that child.

Picture the response of that child, in your memory, as an instantaneous, automatic response of that infant smiling back at you.

Breathe deeply.

Picture and feel that response, which is the warm, simple connection that can occur between two people when they are open to sharing it.

This is the reciprocal loop in its most glorious form. It is you smiling *and* the baby smiling back *and* you returning the smile again that creates the reciprocal loop. This is positive communication in its purest form. No words are spoken, but the exchange of warm regard comes through loud and clear.

Human beings respond to each other in a profound, innate, intuitive way. It is this connection that guides our patterns of communication with one another and goes beyond the spoken word.

The Reciprocal Mirror

Your facial expressions can affect how other people feel. Have you ever stopped to consider how we interpret and understand another person's face? Believe it or not, when we see a face, our eyes receive the information upside down, and to interpret what we see, we first have to turn the picture right side up (Dragoi 2015).

Then, if you are calm and relaxed, another interesting thing happens: when you see a person's face, your own face begins to make movements that mirror it (Dimberg, Thunberg, and Elmehed 2000). Why? It appears that changes in our facial muscles trigger changes in our brains and our emotions. If our facial muscles point downward (typically an indication of sadness), our brains shift and we begin to feel sad; and if we smile, we begin to feel happier. This phenomenon is called *facial feedback* (Kassin, Fein, and Markus 2008). When you look at another person's face, the same feedback process happens: you begin to mirror the expression you see, and then your facial changes activate neurons in your brain that help you decode the experience of your face, and this in turn allows you to interpret what the other person is experiencing. Amazingly, when you look at the expression on someone's face and you begin to mirror it, your facial movements trigger in you the same neural activities it took to produce that expression on the face of the other person (Wood et al. 2015).

All of this neural activity can engender a smoother flow of communication and a sense of genuine connection. We call this process the *reciprocal mirror* because, in essence, the expression you see on the face of the other person is often a reflection of the face you are showing him or her, and vice versa.

Let's take a closer look at the physical cues our faces show and how they affect our communication patterns.

Physical Cues

We are innately attuned to subtle changes in the facial expressions of others (Dimberg, Thunberg, and Elmehed 2000). Even if we see a face for only milliseconds—too short a time to consciously register what we are seeing—our own facial muscles react with distinct patterns that mirror those of the other person's face (Hennenlotter et al. 2009).

The same applies to the feeling of disgust: the brains of people *watching* others who smell a disgusting odor are activated in the same area as the brains of those actually smelling the odor (Wicker et al. 2003). This study indicates that, just by watching another's face, our own brains are stimulated and emotions are automatically triggered.

People who struggle with anxiety often try to gain some control over their emotions by keeping their faces still. Interestingly, research supports the idea that by holding your face still, you may feel less emotion. Researchers showed images of angry and sad faces to two groups of people. In one group, people's faces were free to move as usual, while in the other group, some of the participants' facial muscles had been frozen with Botox. When compared to the non-Botox participants, the people whose faces were free to move showed greater activity in an emotion-generating part of the brain

(Hennenlotter et al. 2009). This indicates that people may experience less emotion when their faces are held still.

Though it may be possible to control some of your anxiety by freezing your face, this comes at a cost. In one creative study, researchers noted that biting down on a pen would immobilize facial muscles related to the expression of happiness. They found that, when compared to people whose faces were free to move, the people whose facial muscles had been immobilized had more difficulty accurately interpreting other people's expressions of happiness (Oberman, Winkielman, and Ramachandran 2007). So if you hold your face still, the lack of movement could interfere with your ability to accurately interpret another person's face and "read" his or her emotional state. It could also make you more prone to misinterpreting what the person is saying.

In Sync

When two people are communicating in person, it's not only their faces that begin to synchronize. They also tend to reflect each other's behaviors, gestures, and breathing patterns, and even their bodies begin to move in rhythm together (Codrons et al. 2014) as their turn-taking activities and rate of speech synchronize (Himberg et al. 2015).

When people reflect each other's physical expressions, they feel more "in sync" with each other; they not only have a better sense of what the other person is feeling, they also feel better about themselves and the other person (Lumsden, Miles, and Macrae 2014). People also feel more compassion toward a person who is mirroring them (Valdesolo and DeSteno 2011). Synchronized activities and movements appear to set a positive foundation for social interaction, creating better cooperation and rapport among the communicators.

Anxiety may also affect synchronization, because if one person is anxious, it may set up a mutual feeling of discomfort. Both may fidget and be vaguely uncomfortable without even knowing why.

Because of this synchronization, it's understandable that relaxation and spontaneity make for an easy flow of communication. A smile can be powerful; seeing another person smile, and smiling back, or even just *thinking* of smiling, triggers a host of positive changes in our nervous systems that creates happy feelings (Barry 2011). But if you suffer from anxiety, even a simple smile can be difficult to muster.

Anxiety can also reduce our ability to feel a connection to our own emotional states and the feelings of others, and can block our intuition in communicating with them. Meditation can help. Kieran Fox and associates, in a review of neuroimaging studies, found that meditation structurally changed and improved the functioning of several areas of the brain associated with emotional self-awareness and other types of awareness (2014).

Having a solid intuitive sense improves your ability to be in tune with and genuinely understand the person with whom you are communicating. The following meditation is designed to strengthen your sense of intuition. The meditation asks you to "look" with your "inner eye." The inner eye is a mystical concept that is said to provide intuition or perception beyond one's visual sight.

KY MEDITATION:
Intuition and Balance
(Bhajan 1998)

Sit in Easy Pose.

Put your thumbs on the mounds of the pinkie finger.

Extend your index finger up and close the other three fingers over the thumb, holding it in place.

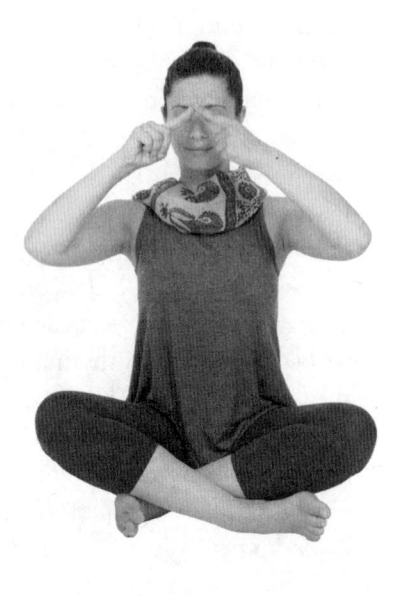

With the right palm facing out and the left palm facing in, touch the pads of the two extended fingers, making a connection between them. They will form an upside-down "V."

Position this ⌃ in front of the "root" (bridge) of the nose, at the point between your eyebrows.

Slowly close your eyes so they are nine-tenths closed, and look at the ⌃ with your inner eye.

With full strength, inhale powerfully through the mouth in two quick sniffs. Each sniff should last 1 second.

Exhale powerfully through the nose in two quick sniffs. Each sniff should last 1 second.

Begin with 1 to 3 minutes, and build to 11 minutes.

To end: Inhale deeply, hold the breath for 20 seconds, and squeeze your body inward.

Exhale like cannon fire.

Inhale deeply, hold for 20 seconds, and put all of your strength into pressing the two extended fingers together. This is said to help balance the central nervous system.

Exhale.

Inhale deeply, hold the breath for 20 seconds, and pressurize all the muscles of the spinal column, one by one, from the tailbone to the highest vertebra (called C1), where the neck connects to the skull.

Exhale and relax.

Inhale and suspend the breath briefly. Exhale and relax the breath, relax the posture.

Throughout your day, try to tap into your intuition and notice any changes in your interactions with others. Being attuned in this way will help improve the way you listen and respond. Positive communication requires an intuitive sense and good listening skills.

Making Healthy Communication a Habit

Healthy communication is a natural exchange with an easy back-and-forth flow of talking and listening. As noted previously, anxiety interferes with communication because it disrupts the natural relay between the speaker and listener. The cues that an anxious person emits can be misread, and the anxious person can also easily misread the cues of the other. *Conscious communication*, as taught by Yogi Bhajan (1999), is a form of non-anxious communication.

Conscious communication suggests that your whole heart, mind, and body become 100 percent involved in the exchange (Bhajan 1999). It begins with being relaxed and alert to the present moment, because in a certain way, authentic, healthy communication is your truth, untarnished by fear and anxiety. Achieving this involves remaining in tune with your intrinsic value, which in turn will express itself in your body by the rhythm of your breathing pattern, your rate of speech, and your way of thinking and speaking.

In healthy communication, we understand ourselves and the other person from a compassionate and neutral place. But sometimes your self-doubt can take over, and you may find yourself being judgmental of yourself or the other person. Being aware of and comfortable with your own positive and negative attributes will improve your ability to tolerate and accept the same in the other person (Bhajan 2006).

When you are speaking, it's important to remember that your words create your future—a compassionate word can uplift someone who is sad, but a harsh word can hurt someone and make matters worse (Bhajan 2006).

When you are listening, it's helpful to stay in the moment, ask questions, and let the other person fully express himself or herself. Although we may think we understand what a person is saying, our own cognitive distortions can make true understanding and acceptance difficult. When you listen, remember that a person may mean something different from what you are hearing. Asking questions for clarification, rather than making assumptions, is typically the best course of action for understanding another's meaning.

Focus on communicating from a mindful and yogic perspective, which does not require the other person to be or say anything. Instead of focusing on what you want from the other person, focus on *you* and *your ability* to stay in an aware but relaxed state. Ask yourself, "Am I relaxed? Am I breathing slowly? Is my posture comfortable and straight? Am I remembering to gently listen?"

Sometimes, even if you achieve a relaxed state, the other person may not always join you there. At those times, it's helpful to remember that you can't control others. Instead, you can exert gentle *self-control* by remaining calm and accepting the person as he or she is, without judgment. This acceptance, though difficult to practice, is the essence of conscious communication.

Once you are interacting in this way, your centered stance serves as an invitation to the other person to meet you in a tranquil state, in his or her own way. Your communication becomes an intuitive, peaceful reciprocal flow. In yogic terms, this back-and-forth is part of a bigger picture: "*Being* itself has a pulse and a sound. A vibration" (Bhajan 1999, 52). With conscious communication, you will feel as if you are a part of this "vibration" of life, and the other person is too.

In Summary

Remember, in every communication with another person, there is a reciprocal feedback loop. Anxiety can interrupt this back-and-forth flow. Increasing your awareness and taking ownership of how you influence the communication you have with others will help you develop healthier and more satisfying relationships. Focusing on what you intend when you are communicating with someone is likely to embed authenticity in the exchange. Healthy communication is more than words. It involves awareness of the feelings and intentions of both people.

Week 5 Daily Y-CBT Practice

Guiding Principle

There is a "reciprocal loop" in all communication. In every encounter between individuals, there is a back-and-forth interaction that creates the mood and the message between the participants. Awareness and ownership of how we influence our interactions is profoundly important in the development of healthy and satisfying relationships.

Yoga and Meditation

Practice the first yoga set, then choose from any of the other three meditations.

1. Set for Heart, Voice, and Intuition

2. Burn Inner Anger

3. Intuition and Balance

4. Heal a Broken Heart

Practice each pose of the yoga set and one of the meditations for a minimum of one minute each.

Daily Living Practice

Take note of your communication patterns this week, and observe how anxiety affects your communication style. Please try out the techniques you learned in this chapter to begin to shift your responses to more centered and confident ones:

*   Observe the reciprocal loop in your daily interactions, and note what you bring to this dynamic.

*   Use the exercises to illuminate your physical and thought reactions to anxiety when you are interacting with others.

*   Practice keeping your intrinsic value in your own pocket when you are having a difficult interaction.

*   Remember to add two new intrinsic values to the list you began last week.

Daily Practice Log

	Sunday		Monday		Tuesday		Wednesday		Thursday		Friday		Saturday	
Time of Day														
	B	A	B	A	B	A	B	A	B	A	B	A	B	A
Yoga/Meditation I Used														
Y-CBT Techniques I Used														

B = Before, A = After

1	2	3	4	5	6	7	8	9	10

Low Anxiety	Moderate Anxiety	High Anxiety

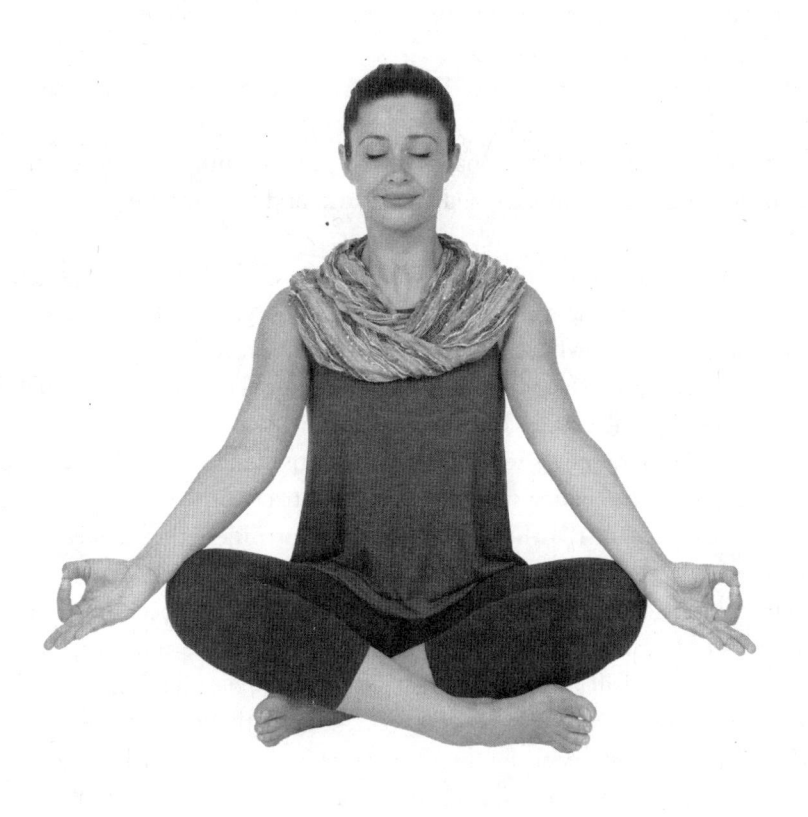

WEEK 6

Developing Radiance

Have you ever noticed that when certain people talk, everyone listens? Another person might voice the same words, but no one pays much attention. Why is that? It has to do with the elusive quality of *radiance*, or *presence*.

When something is radiant, it emits light, it's shining, it's bright, and it glows. When people possess radiance or presence, they are commonly said to be "glowing with happiness" or "bright with confidence and a spark of life." They have charisma or a magnetism that seems to naturally draw other people and good fortune.

The notion of radiance has been part of Eastern thought for a very long time, and recently this idea has surfaced in Western writings. In the yogic way of thinking, radiance is attractive because it is grounded in authenticity and integrity (Bhajan 1999). Two prominent Western authors who have discussed the concept of presence in their many writings and lectures are Amy Cuddy and Eckhart Tolle.

In her book *Presence* (2015), the social psychologist Amy Cuddy writes that people who have presence have a common characteristic: they are attuned to what really matters to them, and this attunement gives them confidence, allowing them to be more comfortable expressing what they feel. Cuddy notes that when we become truly confident and present in the moment, all the elements of our communications—words, facial expressions, and confident body postures—authentically align and support our message. This alignment, she contends, makes us compelling because it creates a powerful connection to our real self, which allows us to honestly connect with others. The combination of personal alignment and attunement to others creates a trustworthiness that makes people more willing to share their real selves in return.

Eckhart Tolle, in *The Power of Now* (1999), uses the word "presence" with an emphasis on the power of staying in the moment. Tolle believes that as you become more tuned in to the present moment in your daily life, you will grow in what he calls *presence power* (Tolle 2013), which he describes as a field of energy around you. He explains that you can grow this field of energy by becoming more and more present in the moment, and by directing your attention inward to neutrally observe your thoughts, your emotions, and how your body is reacting. As you improve your ability to remain aware and calm, even through life's most difficult challenges, this presence power grows.

In yogic theory and practice, the concept of radiance, or presence, is grounded in your awareness of the present moment and in your confident mind-body experience of living in harmony with your values. A radiant person is aligned with himself and attuned to others. This combination creates trust and connection, and encourages authenticity and radiance in other people as well.

This leads us to the guiding principle for this week: ***Our intentions help to focus our attention.*** Several prominent authors have pointed out the benefits of becoming more aware of our intentions, as they often have great influence in our lives (Dyer 2004b; Bhajan 1999; Cuddy 2015). *Intention* is the purpose or attitude that we bring to our interactions with others. Our intentions come from our deepest convictions and values, and when we become aware of these it's easier to focus our *attention* on what really matters to us. This alignment creates an authenticity and a relaxation that generates trust.

Eckhart Tolle refers to the energy field that surrounds you as being a very important element of presence; in yogic terms this field is called the *aura*, and it's a key component in our understanding of radiance. In this way of thinking, radiance is largely considered a function of the brightness and size of your aura. What has for centuries been called the aura or halo can also be spoken of as the electromagnetic field that surrounds you (Bhajan 2003). While the existence of a human aura has never been scientifically proven, the concept is integral to Kundalini Yoga and many world religious traditions. Whether you believe in the human aura or choose to view it as a metaphor, there are meditations focusing on this feature that can enhance the powerful personal quality of radiance.

We will talk more about the concept of the aura shortly, but first here is an exercise to help you better understand what radiance looks and feels like.

EXERCISE:
Think of a Radiant Person

Think of a person you consider radiant. Choose someone you know well or have read about, or perhaps someone you've seen in the media.

Describe his or her style of speaking: _____

_____

Describe this person's posture while seated and while standing: _____

_____

Are this person's words consistent with his or her facial expressions? If so, how?

_____

How do you feel when listening or talking to him or her? _____

_____

The goal of the next question is to discover what you can learn about yourself from watching and interacting with someone who has radiance. Sit up straight and breathe deeply three times. Then ask yourself:

In what ways can I apply my observations of this person to myself?

_____

_____

As you will see next, radiance and anxiety are interrelated: anxiety can interfere with radiance, but radiance can also become a wonderful tool to reduce anxiety.

How Anxiety Interferes with Radiance

Anxiety affects three key elements of radiance: your posture, your mind, and your connection with others.

Posture

A radiant person's body reflects a confident, open attitude. Cuddy explains that people with presence feel confident, secure, and open to others, and this is reflected in their demeanor and posture, which tend to be more relaxed, alert, open, and upright (Cuddy 2015). On the other hand, anxiety often manifests itself in a tense, sometimes slumped posture, and this body language telegraphs a closed and unreceptive attitude.

Mind

A radiant person's mind is conscious and aware in the present moment. In contrast, anxiety takes individuals out of the present; they are more ruminative, worried, and caught up in a kind of self-reflection that shuts out a lot of what's going on around them, further decreasing their confidence.

Connection

A radiant person's interactions are calmer and more attuned to other people because the person's state of mind and body foster connection with others. Because he is more relaxed, a radiant person is authentically more curious and empathic, and he enjoys the company of others.

Anxiety interferes with these qualities and therefore creates problems in communication. Anxiety makes it more difficult to stay in the moment, so an anxious person may not fully hear what others are saying or be able to speak as clearly as she would like; she may feel awkward and "blank" in social situations, adding to her insecurity and physical tension. A tense person's body language may also communicate signals that break the connection with others. She may inadvertently send signals that she is not interested in other people's thoughts and feelings; or she may look as though she wants to end a conversation when actually she just doesn't know what to say.

Simply put, anxiety interferes with radiance because of the many ways it affects one's mind, body, and communications. Here is an exercise that can help you observe this process in yourself.

EXERCISE:
How Anxiety Interferes with Your Radiance

1. Think of a time when you felt on top of your game. Everything was going your way, and you felt very good about yourself.

   Describe your posture: _____

   Did your words match your facial expressions? How so?

   _____

   Describe how you spoke: _____

   How did others respond to you? _____

2. Now, think of a time when you were anxious. What was different?

   Describe your posture: _____

   Did your words match your facial expressions? How so?

   _____

   Describe how you spoke: _____

   How did others respond to you? _____

3. Sit up straight and breathe more deeply and slowly. How can you use what you learned about these two scenarios? Can you see how anxiety reduces your ability to access your own radiance?

   _____

   _____

From this exercise, you can see that anxiety can diminish your radiance and that there's a real difference in the way you feel and the way others respond to you, depending on whether you feel anxious or radiant. The great news is that although radiance is a wonderful, magical quality, it's also a complex of skills. And you can learn it!

Becoming Radiant

How can you develop the skills of radiance? By cultivating a strong awareness of your body and your mind, by developing an understanding of your aura, and by observing how you interact with others.

Many of the Y-CBT techniques you have learned for reducing anxiety also work for developing radiance. For example, before giving a presentation you may feel nervous, but you can still be radiant. You'll feel and appear more radiant if you relax by using the self-calming methods in this book.

Skills of the Body

Radiance creates a glow that begins from within and both accentuates and transcends the physical self. There is a particular beauty that arises from radiance that comes from caring for your physical self and increasing your awareness of your body language. Anyone can become radiant. You too can become radiant by caring for your physical being:

- Develop an awareness of your physical body

- Eat well

- Exercise

- Get enough sleep

- Practice good hygiene

- Wear clothes that express your own style

- Meditate

- Take slow, deep breaths

- Sit and stand straight, expanding your chest and keeping your face, neck, and shoulders relaxed

These are all ways of loving and taking care of yourself, which will increase radiance. Many of these simple ideas are incorporated in the yoga you've been learning throughout this book. With time, as you practice maintaining this more open, confident stance, your mind will follow your body's lead, and you'll begin to feel more self-assured. By learning some new mental skills, you'll be able to fully incorporate this more open attitude into your personality.

Skills of the Mind

The mind of a radiant person is relaxed, attentive, energized, and open. Consider the guiding principle of this chapter: *Our intentions help to focus our attention.* You can hold a gentle intention to become radiant, and, if you keep this intention in mind, you will focus your attention on developing radiance. What you *attend* to has the chance to grow and prosper, while the things you don't pay attention to tend to fall away. A garden provides a good analogy: if you intend to plant a garden, you will begin to envision it and pay a lot of attention to the weather, the soil, the water, and the selection of seeds and plants. Eventually, the garden matures, and you have vegetables or flowers. It's much the same with radiance: if your intention and attention are strong, you'll take actions that will, in time, grow into radiance.

Many of the anxiety-reducing techniques you've learned from this book will help you in your quest to cultivate radiance:

- Notice when your mind is fighting with itself, and take steps to calm it (see The Mind-Body Connection).

- Tune in to the present moment (see The Mind-Body Connection).

- Hold on to your intrinsic value (see Week 4).

- Align your actions with your internal guidance system to create authenticity (see Week 4).

- Practice self-compassion (see Week 4).

- Foster positive interactions with others (see Week 5).

Skills of Radiant Communication

Much of life's joy comes from sharing yourself—your insights and passions, your intellect and spirit—with others.

A natural sense of empathy for others develops in those who have empathy for themselves, and so they are genuinely caring and polite. Wayne Dyer (2004b) refers to people with these qualities as "connectors"—those who genuinely care for others and are able to share their excitement for life. In the presence of such thoughtful people, you may sense an authentic kindness that makes you feel more accepted and more positive about yourself. You may feel calmer, more energized, less isolated, and possibly more inspired to find and develop your own radiance.

Relationship skills come naturally to some but are more difficult for others. Here are several practices that can help you create good communication habits:

- Connect authentically with yourself, which will enable you to connect more easily with others.

- Become aware of your own thoughts, feelings, and reactions.

- Be mindful of the special gifts you have to offer.

- Lean on your intrinsic value.

Building Your Aura

In Kundalini Yoga as taught by Yogi Bhajan, it is believed that everyone is born with a "spark," and if you nurture this light you will become radiant (Bhajan 1999). Practitioners of Kundalini Yoga believe that radiance, in addition to deriving from the elements discussed above, is a function of the brightness and size of your aura. The aura is thought to be the electromagnetic field that surrounds your body.

Hari Kaur Khalsa was sited in the *Yoga Journal* as one of the ten most influential yoga teachers in the United States (Atkins 2016). She explains the aura this way:

> Our bodies are little chemical factories, with many system-operations generating huge amounts of bioelectric activity. Wherever we go, our body continues working, and that process creates an energy that reaches beyond our skin. You can feel this energy, and so can other people! Yogis call this energy the aura.
>
> We all take up space, but when you feel anxious or depressed, you don't feel you deserve to take up space—you try to stay invisible. One of the very basic things that yoga does is, it helps you feel comfortable taking up space. When you exercise or meditate, your posture grows taller, you gain confidence, and your aura grows. This expansion is the basis of why in yoga they say that the aura gives you more confidence, protection and projection (H. K. Khalsa 2016).

From a yogic point of view, when you feel confident, not only do you "grow taller" and feel empowered to occupy your physical space, but your "light" presence may also expand. Confidence and radiance are contained within your aura. The brighter and larger the size of your aura, the more radiance you produce. As Yogi Bhajan explains, "It's the turbine of self-esteem that creates the electromagnetic field" (1989).

To build your aura, you can rely on several of the techniques in this book. Here are some examples:

- Find inspiration in wisdom. As you repeat wise, life-affirming thoughts, aligning your posture and breath with these expansive sentiments, your aura will brighten and grow larger—you'll experience and project radiance. Try these affirmations:

  > *Every moment is an extraordinary, precious event, and I choose to use my energy for excellence while practicing compassion for my human flaws.*
  >
  > *I will practice gratitude, even in the hardest of times.*
  >
  > *I will stand up for what matters to me.*
  >
  > *I will find and enjoy the beauty of every moment, and choose to see the beauty in everyone I meet. In so doing, I will myself emanate beauty.*

- Practice yoga. "Kundalini Yoga is the science of changing and strengthening the radiance to give you an expanded life and greater capacity" (Bhajan 2003, 27).

- Develop a regular meditation practice.

MEDITATION:
To experience your aura

This meditation is said to increase the size and brightness of your aura by developing an awareness of yourself in the space around you.

Sit in Easy Pose with your hands in gyan mudra.

Close your eyes and sit up straight in a comfortable posture.

Bring your attention to your body.

Notice your chest rise and fall as you inhale and exhale deeply through your nose.

Attend to how your body and breath are contained within your skin.

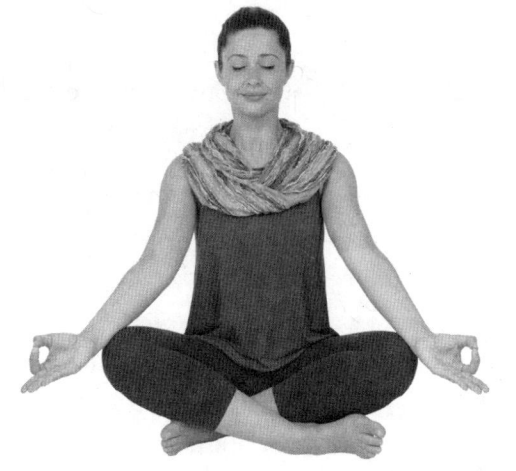

Breathe into your heart center and expand your chest.

Create a visual image of the breath expanding from the heart center outward as you breathe deeply.

Try to feel and picture the air that is just around your body.

Continue to expand your image and breath into the electromagnetic field that surrounds you.

Inhale and suspend the breath briefly. Exhale and relax the breath, relax the posture.

Did you experience a sensation of something that exists beyond your skin? Some people see a light; some people feel an extension of themselves—as though they are larger. If so, you are beginning to sense your aura. If not, don't worry—everyone has an aura, but it can take time and practice to become aware of it. The next meditation uses a breathing technique to increase the size and brightness of the aura. The breath pattern may be unusual for you, so be alert to other new sensations as well.

KY MEDITATION:
Brighten Your Radiance

(Bhajan 2008, 76)

Sit in Easy Pose with your hands in gyan mudra

Close your eyes.

Begin Breath of Fire (see Week 4).

As you become steady and relaxed with the breathing pattern, begin to scan your body.

Feel the pulse of your breath moving through your body.

As you continue to scan your body, do so steadily and with patience and appreciation for the gift of your body.

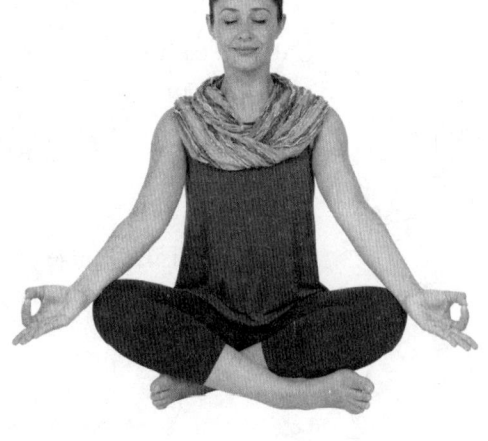

Your attention will guide your breath to every cell of your body.

Stay centered and aware.

As the flow of your breath becomes established, your aura will brighten and grow.

You can visualize light pouring from every pore of your body, extending without limit in every direction.

Begin with 1 minute; you can build to 31 minutes.

Inhale and suspend the breath briefly. Exhale and relax the breath, relax the posture.

In Summary

In this chapter you learned skills to help you develop radiance and enhance your aura. We talked about the ways that anxiety interferes with radiance and how you can use the skills you have learned both to decrease anxiety and to increase radiance. Remember, radiance is a skill you can learn and share with others.

Week 6 and Beyond Daily Y-CBT Practice

Guiding Principle

Our intentions help to focus our attention. The simple act of attending to ourselves—our body, our breath, our thoughts—with nurturing acceptance and encouragement is a powerful mechanism for change. It is important that we come to understand the goals that underlie our thoughts, words, and actions. We are not always conscious of them, and they are critical.

Yoga and Meditation

1. Yoga Warm-Ups for a Flexible Spine (see Week 1)

2. Meditation to experience your aura

3. Brighten Your Radiance

Practice each pose and meditation for a minimum of one minute each.

Daily Living Practice

Your practice this week is to work on expanding your awareness of how you can work with your body and your mind to create a more confident presence, which results in radiance. As you go through each day this week, remind yourself to:

- Notice times when you are anxious: Is there a way to shift your body, breath, and mind to a more confident posture? Practice the exercise How Anxiety Interferes with Your Radiance to help you shift from anxiety to a more confident stance.

- Notice times when everything is going well and you feel confident. Notice your posture, how you are breathing, and what you are thinking. Become more familiar with yourself when you are radiant.

- Add two new qualities to the list of your intrinsic values that you began in Week 4.

After Week 6: Your Daily Y-CBT Practice Log

After you have completed the six-week program, we encourage you to continue your Y-CBT daily practice. You can choose to focus on a topic that is current for you and practice the associated yoga and meditation exercises for a week or longer. In this way, you will continue to deepen your awareness and reinforce the skills that help you to reduce your anxiety and increase your courage, your sense of intrinsic value, and your inner peace.

	Sunday		Monday		Tuesday		Wednesday		Thursday		Friday		Saturday	
Time of Day														
	B	A	B	A	B	A	B	A	B	A	B	A	B	A
Yoga/Meditation I Used														
Y-CBT Techniques I Used														

B = Before, A = After

1	2	3	4	5	6	7	8	9	10
Low Anxiety				Moderate Anxiety				High Anxiety	

Take Your Radiance out into the World

In this book, we have guided you toward managing your anxiety through Y-CBT techniques that reduce fear and increase your ability to respond to challenges with courage, calmness, and awareness of your intrinsic value.

Yogis practice, and they practice a *lot*. Yoga strengthens not just your body but also your mind. Every time you do the yoga poses and meditations, you're relaxing and invigorating your whole physiology—your muscles, your hormones, your nervous system. When you started this book, did you believe that you could actually learn to change and control your responses to stress? Probably not. But now you know that every time you take action to gently control your mind, you are strengthening the skills you need for managing your anxiety. You also now know that, even in the most difficult times, you will be more capable of controlling your reactions. Combining the yogic practice of quieting your mind with the parallel and complementary Y-CBT techniques will continue to help you shift your stress reflexes from tension and worry to a calmer, more focused way of responding.

Life is precious and fragile. Everything can change in a single moment. Allow yourself to slow down and take the time to be grateful for and present to the beauty of life. With practice and patience, you can achieve radiance and a calmer, quieter, less-anxious self.

The beauty of a candle is that it lights the darkness. The beauty of a flower is that it reminds us of the colorful, fragrant magic of life. So it is when you are radiant: without saying a word, your presence brings kindness of heart and energy to the people around you (G. Khalsa 2012). There is a simple peace and magical logic to it all, and the wonder is, these are skills you can learn.

We hope this book has helped you on your journey to a more relaxed and open life, and that it has brought you relief from anxiety and inspired you to grow. We wish you continued success and all the best that life has to give.

APPENDIX

Attending a Kundalini Yoga Class

If you want to attend a yoga class in your area, you will likely find many styles, sizes, and speeds to choose from. There really is a yoga class for everyone, and the funnest part of the experience can be in shopping around.

Yoga centers often offer special rates for beginners, so you can sample a variety of classes until you find one that suits you. You'll want to start with a beginner's or "gentle" class. Although the yoga in this book is designed to be easy, yoga classes at studios can be quite strenuous. Most people find that a particular teacher or style of yoga suits them better than others.

In the United States, you'll find Kundalini Yoga classes in almost every state. You'll also find Kundalini Yoga classes all over the world, including in Europe, Russia, South America, China, Israel, Egypt, Africa, and Australia.

If you find a gentle or beginner's Kundalini Yoga class near you, here's what the class will likely be like:

- When you walk in, you'll find people sitting on blankets or yoga mats, often with their legs crossed. If you need a chair, you can ask for one ahead of time.

- As the class starts, you'll be asked to sit up straight and bring your hands together at the center of your chest. You'll begin with a deep breath, followed by a mantra: "*Ong Namo Guru Dev Namo.*" This mantra is said to tune you in to the teacher within you and is chanted before you begin any Kundalini Yoga or meditation. You can hear it here: https://www.3ho.org/files/mp3s /adi-mantra.mp3.

- After the mantra, you'll do about a half hour of yoga, followed by a relaxation sequence or a meditation, or both. These classes can be musical, and you'll hear songs and mantras in English and in an ancient Indian language.

Acknowledgments

We would like to express our gratitude to Riverside Community Care for serving as a home for Y-CBT. We are grateful for the support with the research and the opportunity to grow the Y-CBT project at Riverside. We are most appreciative of the many people we have known whose journeys through their struggles with anxiety have afforded us the opportunity to learn and develop this model. Thank you to the interns at Riverside who helped with the research, and to our friends who reviewed and supported our work: Savitri Kaur Khalsa, Casey Strumpf, Felicia Buebel, Siri Sevak Kaur Khalsa, Carolynne D'Agostino, and Marcel Descheneaux. Many thanks to John Boisseau DNP, for offering his consultation and expertise with the material on physiology. Our deep appreciation goes to Siri Neel Kaur Khalsa and the Kundalini Research Institute for all of the support and wisdom. Special thanks to Elizabeth Hollis Hanson, Clancy Drake, and the New Harbinger editorial staff who worked with us throughout the development of this book.

References

American Psychiatric Association. 2013. *Diagnostic and Statistical Manual of Mental Disorders*. 5th ed. Arlington, VA: American Psychiatric Publishing.

Atkins, A. 2016. "10 Influential Teachers Who Have Shaped Yoga in America." *Yoga Journal*, February 8. http://www.yogajournal.com/slideshow/10-influential-teachers-shaped-yoga-america/#8.

Barlow, D., and M. Craske. 2007. *Mastery of Your Anxiety and Panic*. Oxford: Oxford University Press.

Barry, S. R. 2011. "I Feel Your Smile, I Feel Your Pain." *Psychology Today*, February 7. https://www.psychologytoday.com/blog/eyes-the-brain/201102/i-feel-your-smile-i-feel-your-pain.

Beck, J. S. 1995. *Cognitive Behavioral Therapy: Basics and Beyond*. New York: Guildford Press.

Bhajan, Y. 1970. "Living in Love." Lecture, Española, NM, June. https://www.3ho.org/kundalini-yoga/yogi-bhajan-lecture-living-love.

——. 1983a. *Kundalini Yoga for Youth and Joy*. Española, NM: Kundalini Research Institute.

——. 1983b. Lecture, Berkeley, CA, September 28.

——. 1985. Lecture, Mexico City, Mexico, April 28.

——. 1989. Lecture, Rome, Italy, May 26.

——. 1991. Lecture, Los Angeles, CA, November 18. Also in Khalsa, H. 1994. *Physical Wisdom: Kundalini Yoga as Taught by Yogi Bhajan*. Española, NM: Kundalini Research Institute.

——. 1992. Lecture, December 31.

——. 1995. Lecture, December 27. Also in Bhajan, Y., and H. K. Khalsa. 2006. *Praana, Praanee, Praanayam: Exploring the Breath Technology of Kundalini Yoga as Taught by Yogi Bhajan*. Española, NM: Kundalini Research Institute.

——. 1997. Lecture, March 25.

——. 1998. Lecture, June 3. Also in Bhajan, Y., and H. K. Khalsa. 2006. *Praana, Praanee, Praanayam: Exploring the Breath Technology of Kundalini Yoga as Taught by Yogi Bhajan*, edited by H. K. Khalsa. Española, NM: Kundalini Research Institute.

——. 1999. *Conscious Communications: KRI International Teacher Training Certification Level 2 Module*. Española, NM: Kundalini Research Institute.

——. 2000. Lecture, San Diego, CA, April 15.

——. 2003. *KRI International Teacher Training Manual Level 1*. Española, NM: Kundalini Research Institute.

——. 2006. *Authentic Relationships: KRI International Teacher Training Certification Level 2 Practitioner Certification Course*. Española, NM: Kundalini Research Institute.

————. 2008. *Vitality and Stress: KRI International Teacher Training Certification Level 2 Module*. Española, NM: Kundalini Research Institute.

————. 2009. *I Am a Woman: Creative, Sacred & Invincible—Essential Kriyas for Women in the Aquarian Age*. Española, NM: Kundalini Research Institute.

Bhajan, Y., and G. S. Khalsa. 1998. *The Mind: Its Projections and Multiple Facets*. Española, NM: Kundalini Research Institute.

Bhajan, Y., and H. K. Khalsa. 2000. *Self-Experience Kundalini Yoga as Taught by Yogi Bhajan*. Española, NM: Kundalini Research Institute.

————. 2006. *Praana, Praanee, Praanayam: Exploring the Breath Technology of Kundalini Yoga as Taught by Yogi Bhajan*, edited by H. K. Khalsa. Española, NM: Kundalini Research Institute.

Borkovec, T. D., M. Newman, A. Pincus, and R. Lytle. 2002. "A Component Analysis of Cognitive-Behavioral Therapy for Generalized Anxiety Disorder and the Role of Interpersonal Problems." *Journal of Consulting and Clinical Psychology* 70: 288–298.

Bourne, E. 2015. *The Anxiety and Phobia Workbook*. 6th ed. Oakland, CA: New Harbinger Publications.

Breines, J. G., and S. Chen. 2012. "Self-Compassion Increases Self-Improvement Motivation." *Personality and Social Psychology Bulletin* 38: 1133–1143.

Broyd, S. J., C. Demanuele, S. Debener, S. K. Helps, C. J. James, and E. J. Sonuga-Barke. 2009. "Default-Mode Brain Dysfunction in Mental Disorders: A Systematic Review." *Neuroscience and Biobehavioral Reviews* 33: 279–296.

Cabral, L. F., T. C. D'Elia, D. S. Marins, W. A. Zin, and F. S. Guimarães. 2015. "Pursed Lip Breathing Improves Exercise Tolerance in COPD: A Randomized Crossover Study." *European Journal of Physical and Rehabilitation Medicine* 51: 79–88.

Chapman, I. M. 2016. "Introduction to Pituitary Disorders." Merck Manual Professional Version. https://www.merckmanuals.com/professional/endocrine-and-metabolic-disorders/pituitary-disorders/introduction-to-pituitary-disorders.

Codrons, E., N. F. Bernardi, M. Vandoni, and L. Bernardi. 2014. "Spontaneous Group Synchronization of Movements and Respiratory Rhythms." *PLoS ONE* 9: e107538.

Collins, A., and E. Koechlin. 2012. "Reasoning, Learning, and Creativity: Frontal Lobe Function and Human Decision-Making. *PLoS Biology* 10: e1001293.

Covey, S. T. 1989. *The 7 Habits of Highly Effective People: Powerful Lessons in Personal Change*. 1st Fireside ed. New York: Simon & Schuster.

Covey, S. T. 1992. *Principle Centered Leadership*. 1st Fireside ed. New York: Simon & Schuster.

Critchley, H. D. 2009. "Psychophysiology of Neural, Cognitive and Affective Integration: fMRI and Autonomic Indicants." *International Journal of Psychophysiology* 73: 88–94. Retrieved from http://doi.org/10.1016/j.ijpsycho.2009.01.012.

Cuddy, A. 2015. *Presence: Bringing Your Boldest Self to Your Biggest Challenges*. New York: Little, Brown.

Daubenmier, J., J. Sze, C. Kerr, M. Kemeny, and W. Mehling. 2013. "Follow Your Breath: Respiratory Interoceptive Accuracy in Experienced Meditators." *Psychophysiology* 50: 777–789.

De Bruin, E. I., van der Zwan, J. E., & S. M. Bögels. 2016. "A RCT Comparing Daily Mindfulness Meditations, Biofeedback Exercises, and Daily Physical Exercise on Attention Control, Executive Functioning, Mindful

Awareness, Self-Compassion, and Worrying in Stressed Young Adults." *Mindfulness* 7(5): 1182–1192. http://doi.org/10.1007/s12671-016-0561-5.

Desikachar, T. K. V. 1995. *The Heart of Yoga: Developing a Personal Practice.* Rochester, VT: Inner Traditions.

Dimberg, U., M. Thunberg, and K. Elmehed. 2000. "Unconscious Facial Reactions to Emotional Facial Expressions." *American Psychological Society* 11:86–89.

Dimitriev, D. A., E. V. Saperova, and A. D. Dimitriev. 2016. "State Anxiety and Nonlinear Dynamics of Heart Rate Variability in Students." *PLoS ONE* 11: e0146131.

Dusek, J., and H. Benson. 2009. "Mind-Body Medicine: A Model of the Comparative Clinical Impact of the Acute Stress and Relaxation Responses." *Minnesota Medicine.* 92:47–50.

Dyer, W. W. 2004a. *Staying on the Path.* Carlsbad, CA: Hay House.

Dyer, W. W. 2004b. *The Power of Intention: Learning to Co-create Your World Your Way.* Carlsbad, CA: Hay House.

Evans, S., S. Ferrando, M. Findler, C. Stowell, C. Smart, and D. Haglin. 2008. "Mindfulness-Based Cognitive Therapy for Generalized Anxiety Disorder." *Journal of Anxiety Disorders* 22: 716–721.

Feuerstein, G. 2008. *The Yoga Tradition: Its History, Literature, Philosophy and Practice.* Chino Valley, AZ: Hohm Press.

Field, T. 2011. "Yoga Clinical Research Review." *Complementary Therapies in Clinical Practice* 17: 1–8.

Fox, K., S. Nijeboer, M. Dixon, J. Floman, M. Ellamil, and S. Rumak. 2014. "Is Meditation Associated with Altered Brain Structure? A Systematic Review and Meta-Analysis of Morphometric Neuroimaging in Meditation Practitioners." *Neuroscience and Biobehavioral Reviews* 43: 48–73.

Gard, T., J. Noggle, C. Par, D. Vago, and A. Wilson. 2014. "Potential Self-Regulatory Mechanisms of Yoga for Psychological Health." *Frontiers in Human Neuroscience* 8 (article 770).

Goleman, D. 1995. *Emotional Intelligence: Why It Can Matter More Than IQ.* New York: Bantam Books.

Goleman, D. 2004. *Primal Leadership: Learning to Lead with Emotional Intelligence.* Boston: Harvard Business School Press.

Greenberger, D., and C. Padesky. 1995. *Mind Over Mood: Change How You Feel by Changing the Way You Think.* New York: Guilford Press.

Hasenkamp, W., C. D. Wilson-Mendenhall, E. Duncan, and L. W. Barsalou 2012. "Mind Wandering and Attention During Focused Meditation: A Fine-Grained Temporal Analysis of Fluctuating Cognitive States." *Neuroimage* 59: 750–760.

Hay, L. L. 2004. *Love Yourself, Heal Your Life.* Carlsbad, CA: Hay House.

Hennenlotter, A., C. Dresel, F. Castrop, A. Ceballos-Baumann, M. Afra, A. Wohlschläger, and B. Haslinger. 2009. "The Link Between Facial Feedback and Neural Activity Within Central Circuitries of Emotion—New Insights from Botulinum Toxin-Induced Denervation of Frown Muscles." *Cerebral Cortex* 19: 537–42.

Himberg, T., L. Hirvenkari, A. Mandel, and R. Hari. 2015. "Word-by-Word Entrainment of Speech Rhythm During Joint Story Building." *Frontiers in Psychology* 6: 797.

Hoffman, D. L., E. M. Dukes, and H. U. Wittchen. 2008. "Human and Economic Burden of Generalized Anxiety Disorder." *Depression and Anxiety* 25: 72–90.

Hofmann, S. G., and J. A. Smits. 2008. "Cognitive-Behavioral Therapy for Adult Anxiety Disorders: A Meta-Analysis of Randomized Placebo-Controlled Trials." *Journal of Clinical Psychiatry* 69: 621–632.

Hofmann, S. G., Sawyer, A. T., Witt, A. A., & D. Oh. 2010. The Effect of Mindfulness-based Therapy on Anxiety and Depression: A Meta-analytic Review. *Journal of Consulting and Clinical Psychology* 78(2): 169–183. doi:10.1037/a0018555.

Hollis-Walker, L., and K. Colosimo. 2011. "Mindfulness, Self-Compassion, and Happiness in Non-Meditators: A Theoretical And Empirical Examination." *Personality and Individual Differences* 50: 223–227.

Jerath, R., Crawford, M. W., Barnes, V. A., & K. Harden. 2015. "Self-Regulation of Breathing as a Primary Treatment for Anxiety." *Appl Psychophysiol Biofeedback* 40: 107. doi:10.1007/s10484-015-9279-8.

Jindani, F., N. Turner, and S. B. Khalsa. 2015. "A Yoga Intervention for Posttraumatic Stress: A Preliminary Randomized Control Trial." *Journal of Evidence-Based Complementary and Alternative Medicine* 2015: 351746. doi:10.1155/2015/351746.

Kassin, S., S. Fein, and H. Markus. 2008. *Social Psychology.* 7th ed. Boston: Houghton Mifflin.

Kessler R. C., W. T. Chiu, O. Demler, and E. E. Walters. 2005a. "Lifetime Prevalence and Age-of-Onset Distributions of *DSM-IV* Disorders in the National Comorbidity Survey Replication." *Archives of General Psychiatry* 62: 593–602.

Kessler R. C., W. T. Chiu, O. Demler, and E. E. Walters. 2005b. "Prevalence, Severity, and Comorbidity of 12-Month *DSM-IV* Disorders in the National Comorbidity Survey Replication." *Archives of General Psychiatry* 62: 617–627.

Khalsa, G. 2012. *The 21 Stages of Meditation.* Santa Cruz, NM: Kundalini Research Institute.

Khalsa, H. 1994. *Physical Wisdom: Kundalini Yoga as Taught by Yogi Bhajan.* Española, NM: Kundalini Research Institute.

Khalsa, H. K. 2015. Personal communication, September.

Khalsa, H. K. 2016. Personal communication, April.

Khalsa, H. K., and M. Seibel. 2002. *A Woman's Book of Yoga.* New York: Penguin Group.

Khalsa, M. K., J. M. Greiner-Ferris, and J. Boisseau. Forthcoming. "Yoga-CBT (Y-CBT) for the Treatment of Anxiety and Depression."

Khalsa, M. K., J. M. Greiner-Ferris, S. G. Hofmann, and S. B. S. Khalsa. 2014. "Yoga-Enhanced Cognitive Behavioural Therapy (Y-CBT) for Anxiety Management: A Pilot Study." *Clinical Psychology and Psychotherapy* 22: 364–371.

Khalsa, S. B., and S. Cope. 2006. "Effects of a Yoga Lifestyle Intervention on Performance-Related Characteristics of Musicians: A Preliminary Study." *Medical Science Monitor* 12: 325–331.

Khalsa, S. B., S. M. Shorter, S. Cope, G. Wyshak, and E. Sklar. 2009. "Yoga Ameliorates Performance Anxiety and Mood Disturbance in Young Professional Musicians." *Applied Psychophysiology and Biofeedback* 34: 279–289.

Khalsa, S. B. S. 2004. "Yoga as a Therapeutic Intervention: A Bibliometric Analysis of Published Research Studies." *Indian Journal of Physiology and Pharmacology* 48: 269–285.

Khalsa, S. N. K. 2014. Personal communication, December.

Khalsa, S. P. K. 2007. *Kundalini Yoga Sadhana Guidelines.* 2nd ed. Santa Cruz, NM: Kundalini Research Institute.

Kirkwood, G., H. Rampes, V. Tuffrey, J. Richardson, and K. Pilkington. 2005. "Yoga for Anxiety: A Systematic Review of the Research Evidence." *British Journal of Sports Medicine* 39: 884–891.

Knaus, W. 2014. *The Cognitive Behavioral Workbook for Anxiety: A Step-By-Step Program.* Oakland, CA: New Harbinger Publications.

Krieger, T., D. Altenstein, I. Baettig, N. Doerig, and M. G. Holtforth. 2013. "Self-Compassion in Depression: Associations with Depressive Symptoms, Rumination and Avoidance in Depressed Patients." *Behavior Therapy* 44: 501–513.

Li, P., and J. Stamatakis. 2011. "What Happens in the Brain When We Experience a Panic Attack?" *Scientific American*, July 1. http://www.scientificamerican.com/article/what-happens-in-the-brain-when-we -experience/.

Lumsden J., L. K. Miles, and C. N. Macrae. 2014. "Sync or Sink? Interpersonal Synchrony Impacts Self-Esteem." *Frontiers in Psychology* 5: 1064.

Lutz, A., H. A. Slagter, J. D. Dunne, and R. J. Davidson. 2008. "Attention Regulation and Monitoring in Meditation." *Trends in Cognitive Science* 12: 163–169.

Mehrabian, A., and J. S. Blum. 1997. "Physical Appearance, Attractiveness, and the Mediating Role of Emotions." *Current Psychology* 16: 20–41.

Meuret A. E., F. H. Wilhelm, T. Ritz, W. T. Roth. 2008. "Feedback of End-Tidal pCO2 As a Therapeutic Approach for Panic Disorder." *Journal of Psychiatric Research* 42: 560–568.

Neff, K. D. 2003. "The Development and Validation of a Scale to Measure Self-Compassion." *Self and Identity* 2: 223–250.

Neff, K. D., K. L. Kirkpatrick, and S. S. Rude. 2007. "An Examination of Self-Compassion in Relation to Positive Psychological Functioning and Personality Traits." *Journal of Research in Personality* 41: 908–916.

Newmark, T. 2012. "Cases in Visualization for Improved Athletic Performance." *Psychiatric Annals* 42: 385–387.

Norton, P. J., and E. C. Price. 2007. "A Meta-Analytic Review of Adult Cognitive-Behavioral Treatment Outcome Across the Anxiety Disorders." *Journal of Nervous and Mental Disease* 195: 521–531.

Oberman, L., P. Winkielman, and V. Ramachandran. 2007. "Face to Face: Blocking Facial Mimicry Can Selectively Impair Recognition of Emotional Expressions." *Social Neuroscience* 2: 167–178.

Paulus, M. P. 2013. "The Breathing Conundrum: Interception Sensitivity and Anxiety." *Depression and Anxiety* 30: 315–320.

Peng, C. K., J. E. Mietus, Y. Liu, G. Khalsa, P. S. Douglas, H. Benson et al. 1999. "Exaggerated Heart Rate Oscillations During Two Meditation Techniques." *International Journal of Cardiology* 70: 101–107.

Raes, F. 2010. "Rumination and Worry as Mediators of the Relationship Between Self-Compassion and Depression and Anxiety." *Personality and Individual Differences* 48: 757–761.

Roth, W. 2005. "Physiological Markers for Anxiety: Panic Disorder and Phobias." *International Journal of Psychophysiology* 58: 190–197.

Segal, Z. V., J. M. Williams, and J. D. Teasdale. 2002. *Mindfulness-Based Cognitive Therapy for Depression.* New York: Guilford Press.

Shannahoff-Khalsa, D. S. 2004. "An Introduction to Kundalini Yoga Meditation Techniques That Are Specific for the Treatment of Psychiatric Disorders." *Journal of Alternative and Complementary Medicine* 10: 91–101.

Shapiro, D., I. A. Cook, D. M. Davydov, C. Ottaviani, A. F. Leuchter, and M. Abrams. 2007. "Yoga as a Complementary Treatment of Depression: Effects of Traits and Moods on Treatment Outcome." *Journal of Evidence-Based Complementary Alternative Medicine* 4: 493–502.

Spicuzza, L., A. Gabutti, C. Porta, N. Montano, and L. Bernardi. 2000. "Yoga and Chemoreflex Response to Hypoxia and Hypercapnia." *Lancet* 356: 1,495–1,496.

Stahl, S. 2008. *Stahl's Essential Psychopharmacology: Neuroscientific Basis and Practical Application.* 3rd ed. New York: Cambridge University Press.

Streeter, C. C., P. L. Gerbarg, R. B. Saper, D. A. Ciraulo, R. P. Brown. 2012. "Effects of Yoga on the Autonomic Nervous System, Gamma-Aminobutyric-Acid, and Allostasis in Epilepsy, Depression, and Post-Traumatic Stress Disorder." *Medical Hypotheses* 78: 571–579.

Streeter, C. C., T. H. Whitfield, L. Owen, T. Rein, S. K. Karri, A. Yakhkind, and J. E. Jensen. 2010. "Effects of Yoga Versus Walking on Mood, Anxiety, and Brain GABA Levels: A Randomized Controlled MRS Study." *Journal of Alternative and Complementary Medicine* 16: 1145–1152.

Taylor, V. A., J. Grant, V. Daneault, G. Scavone, E. Breton, S. Roffe-Vidal, J. Courtemanche, A. Lavarenne, and M. Beauregard. 2011. "Impact of Mindfulness on the Neural Responses to Emotional Pictures in Experienced and Beginner Meditators." *Neuroimage* 57: 1524–1533.

Tolle, E. 1999. *The Power of Now: A Guide to Spiritual Enlightenment.* Novato, CA: New World Library; Vancouver, BC: Namaste Publishing.

Tolle, E. 2013. "Creating Consciousness to Grow in Presence Power." In *The Power of Now: A Guide to Spiritual Enlightenment.* Novato, CA: New World Library; Vancouver, BC: Namaste Publishing. Retrieved from http://communicate.eckharttolle.com/news/2013/07/12/creating-consciousness-to-grow-in-presence -power/.

Tsuchitani, C. 2015. "Visual Processing: Eye and Retina." In *Neuroscience Online: The Open-Access Neuroscience Electronic Textbook.* McGovern Medical School at UTHealth. http://neuroscience.uth.tmc.edu/s2/chapter 14.html.

Valdesolo, P., and D. DeSteno. 2011. "Synchrony and the Social Tuning of Compassion." *Emotion,* 11: 262–266.

Van Dam, N. T., S. C. Sheppard, J. P. Forsyth, and M. Earleywine. 2011. "Self-Compassion Is a Better Predictor Than Mindfulness of Symptom Severity and Quality of Life in Mixed Anxiety." *Journal of Anxiety Disorders* 25: 123–130.

Watts V. 2016. "Kundalini Yoga Found to Enhance Cognitive Functioning in Older Adults." *Psychiatric News,* May 3. http://psychnews.psychiatryonline.org/doi/full/10.1176/appi.pn.2016.4b11#.VzIhfT_2e10.facebook.

Wicker, B., C. Keysers, J. Plailly, J. P. Royet, V. Gallese, and G. Rizzolatti. 2003. "Both of Us Disgusted in My Insula: The Common Neural Basis of Seeing and Feeling Disgust." *Neuron* 40: 655–664.

Wood, A., G. Lupyan, S. Sherrin, and P. Niedenthal. 2015. "Altering Sensorimotor Feedback Disrupts Visual Discrimination of Facial Expressions." *Psychonomic Bulletin and Review,* November 5.

Julie Greiner-Ferris, LICSW, has over twenty-five years of experience in the treatment of mental health issues. A graduate of Boston College School of Social Work, she is cocreator of yoga-cognitive behavioral therapy (Y-CBT), and is currently program director of outpatient services at Riverside Community Care in Upton, MA.

Manjit Kaur Khalsa, EdD, is cocreator of Y-CBT. An experienced psychologist, she practices at Riverside Community Care in Upton, MA, and has a private practice in Millis, MA. She is a longtime Kundalini yoga teacher, student of Yogi Bhajan, and president of Sikh Dharma of Massachusetts—the corporation which oversees the Guru Ram Das Ashram in Millis, MA.

FROM OUR PUBLISHER—

As the publisher at New Harbinger and a clinical psychologist since 1978, I know that emotional problems are best helped with evidence-based therapies. These are the treatments derived from scientific research (randomized controlled trials) that show what works. Whether these treatments are delivered by trained clinicians or found in a self-help book, they are designed to provide you with proven strategies to overcome your problem.

Therapies that aren't evidence-based—whether offered by clinicians or in books—are much less likely to help. In fact, therapies that aren't guided by science may not help you at all. That's why this New Harbinger book is based on scientific evidence that the treatment can relieve emotional pain.

This is important: if this book isn't enough, and you need the help of a skilled therapist, use the following resources to find a clinician trained in the evidence-based protocols appropriate for your problem. And if you need more support—a community that understands what you're going through and can show you ways to cope—resources for that are provided below, as well.

Real help is available for the problems you have been struggling with. The skills you can learn from evidence-based therapies will change your life.

Matthew McKay, PhD
Publisher, New Harbinger Publications

**If you need a therapist, the following organization
can help you find a therapist trained in cognitive behavioral therapy (CBT).**

The Association for Behavioral & Cognitive Therapies (ABCT) Find-a-Therapist service offers a list of therapists schooled in CBT techniques. Therapists listed are licensed professionals who have met the membership requirements of ABCT and who have chosen to appear in the directory.
Please visit www.abct.org and click on *Find a Therapist*.

**For additional support for patients, family, and friends,
please contact the following:**

Anxiety and Depression Association of American (ADAA)
please visit www.adaa.org

National Alliance on Mental Illness (NAMI)
please visit www.nami.org

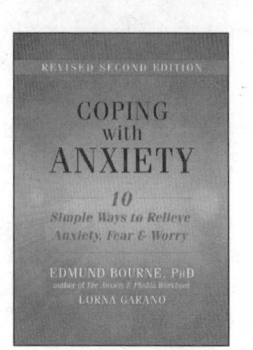
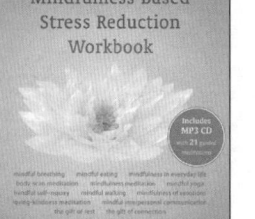
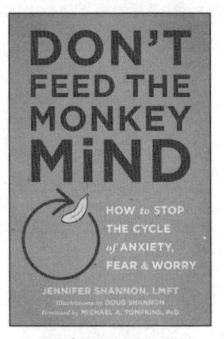
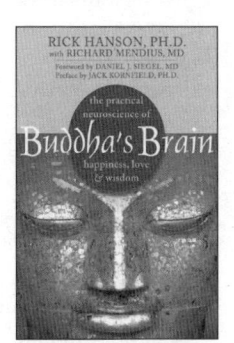